Twelve-Lead Electrocardiography

Second Edition

D. Bruce Foster

Twelve-Lead Electrocardiography

Theory and Interpretation

Second Edition

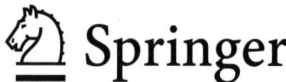 Springer

D. Bruce Foster, DO
Department of Emergency Medicine
Waynesboro Hospital
and
Pennsylvania Institute of Applied Health Sciences
Waynesboro, PA, 17268
USA

British Library Cataloguing in Publication Data
Foster, D. Bruce, 1945–
    Twelve-lead electrocardiography : theory and
    interpretation. – 2nd ed.
    1. Electrocardiography
    I. Title II. Foster, D. Bruce, 1945–. Twelve-lead
    electrocardiography for ACLS providers
    616.1'2'07547
ISBN-13: 9781846285929
ISBN-10: 1846285925

Library of Congress Control Number: 2006932407

ISBN-10: 1-84628-592-5   e-ISBN-10: 1-84628-610-7
ISBN-13: 978-1-84628-592-9   e-ISBN-13: 978-1-84628-610-0

Printed on acid-free paper

© Springer-Verlag London Limited 2007

Originally Published as *Twelve-Lead Electrocardiography for ACLS Providers*, WB Saunders, Co.,
1996. ISBN 0721658733.

9 8 7 6 5 4 3 2 1

Springer Science+Business Media
springer.com

To those delightful little souls who daily make me smile:
Mckenzie, Lleyton, Alexa, and Olivia.

Foreword

If you are a cardiologist or have a photographic memory, you may not need Dr. Foster's new book. But, for the rest of us on the front lines of emergency care, it is a valuable resource that you will want to have by your side at work. I have had the first edition of this book by my station in the emergency department for ten years now. I use it everyday for teaching house staff and often turn to it for reference myself.

For those of us without perfect memories, Dr. Foster's clinical approach is ideal. He has the knack of making the complex simple. He does not expect the reader to memorize every squiggle on the page; instead he inspires understanding by giving readers the tools they need to comprehend why ECGs look the way they do. When a resident comes to me with an ECG, I do not have to spend ten minutes delivering a confusing explanation. I just open Dr. Foster's book to the right page and hand it to the resident for review.

The book is organized so that you can turn to the relevant chapter and instantly know what the differential diagnosis might be. His selection of case studies covers the vast majority of the ECGs you will be called on to read in any sort of emergent situation; anything else can wait for the cardiologist.

This second edition features some extensively revised new chapters that make it even more useful than the first. Three very clinical chapters, in particular, offer a roadmap to your daily practice. Chapter 9 gives an excellent summary of the pitfalls that can plague a physician in diagnosing infarctions. Chapter 10 provides a concise, coherent review of anginal syndromes that makes it possible for the novice to catch on quickly. And the case presentations in Chapter 14 offer a spectrum of fascinating real-life clinical scenarios that help you to integrate the ECG into daily clinical practice and structure your approach to acute coronary syndromes. They also serve to show us all why an ECG is but one of the many clues that must ultimately be synthesized into an accurate diagnosis.

Mark L. Feldman, MD
Supervising Physician
Emergency Department
Whangarei Base Hospital
Whangarei, New Zealand

Preface

Ten years have passed since *Twelve Lead Electrocardiography for ACLS Providers* was written in response to a need for a clear, concise, introductory level text on the morphologic interpretation of electrocardiograms. This need has grown more compelling in the last decade, as a multiplicity of efficacious therapeutic interventions has made the early recognition of acute coronary syndromes ever more important. The text was developed primarily for physicians, physicians' assistants, nurses, and paramedics who are advanced cardiac life support (ACLS) certified and are already familiar with cardiac dysrhythmias. Therefore, the text deals solely with morphology and does not discuss dysrhythmias.

The need for the first edition was initially spurred by the revolutionary development in the 1980s of thrombolytic therapy for acute myocardial infarction (AMI), and, subsequently, the evolution of percutaneous coronary intervention. The availability of these tools, and their time dependency, has magnified the critical role of first responders and primary care providers in the early recognition and treatment of AMI.

The clinical chapters in this second edition have been extensively rewritten to reflect new concepts in the clinical classification of patients with chest pain, including acute coronary syndrome, and ST and non–ST-segment elevation myocardial infarction. Sections have been added on the diagnosis of AMI in patients with bundle branch block (BBB), and the case presentations have been expanded and updated to better reflect contemporary practice. Additional illustrations and new references have been incorporated.

I have tried to include all of the pertinent information that ACLS providers working in EMS systems, primary care centers, emergency departments, and critical care units will need to know to implement chest pain evaluation protocols and, hopefully, to speed coronary intervention.

In reality, however, the text has proven to be equally valuable to medical students and non-critical care physicians who need a working knowledge of the important fundamentals of morphologic electrocardiography, but who need not become professional electrocardiographers. Thus, the text emphasizes simplicity, clinically useful concepts, and common clinical parlance. It is written in a conversational tone, and is not intended to serve as a reference text for serious postgraduate students of electrocardiography.

Nevertheless, fundamental electrophysiologic principles are emphasized to the extent that students have the opportunity to deduce patterns created by both physiologic and pathologic processes, rather than relying on memorizing electrocardiographic (ECG) patterns of disease. I have tried to communicate the sense of joy that comes from deduction and understanding, as opposed to the drudgery of memorization.

There are many people who played an important role in the writing of this text, primary among whom are the many students who have instructed me in what works and what doesn't over 15 years of teaching electrocardiography. This second edition is my thanks for the joy they have shared with me in learning.

And finally, special thanks go, again, to Lauren Datcher, R.N., whose eagle eyes never fail to defect virtually every one of my ubiquitous manuscript errors.

D. Bruce Foster, DO

Contents

Essential Cardiac Anatomy and Physiology as It Relates to the Electrocardiogram

Developing the capability of interpreting a 12-lead electrocardiogram depends upon an understanding of a few fundamental principles of anatomy and physiology. In this chapter, I will review the electrical conduction system of the heart and the methods that are used to record depolarization.

The Specialized Cardiac Conduction System

In the normal heart during sinus rhythm, impulse formation is initiated in the *sinoatrial (SA) node* (Figure 1.1), and then spreads as a wave of depolarization over the atria until it reaches the *atrioventricular (AV) node*, which is near the junction of the interatrial and interventricular septa.

The AV node represents the sole pathway for conducting the impulse from the atria to the ventricles, except when it is bypassed by abnormal congenital pathways. Its unique purpose is to slow the rate of impulse conduction to give the atria time to finish emptying of blood and the ventricles time to finish filling with blood. This is necessary because mechanical contraction of cardiac muscle is normally slower than the rapid process of electrical depolarization (Figure 1.2).

The *common bundle of His* next conducts the impulse through the superior ventricular septum and then quickly divides into the *right and left bundle branch* (Figure 1.1). Perhaps because the left ventricle is bigger than the right ventricle, the left bundle splits into two *hemibundles*, one running anteriorly and superiorly out of the page toward the reader, and the other running posteriorly and inferiorly into the page, as if away from the reader.

Finally, the bundle branches divide numerous times into *Purkinje fibers*, which are the final pathway for conduction of the impulse to ventricular muscle. Once ventricular muscle is stimulated by the impulse traveling down the Purkinje fibers, it depolarizes outwardly from *endocardium* to *epicardium*.

Electrical impulses are conducted much more rapidly through the specialized conduction system of the heart described in the previous paragraphs than through typical cardiac muscle. This allows the electrical impulse to reach almost all ventricular muscles nearly simultaneously, thus, allowing for

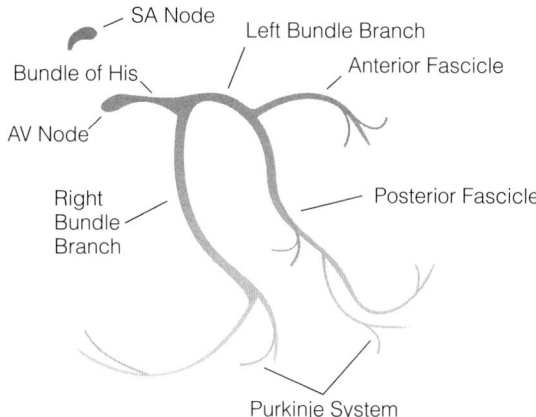

Figure 1.1. The specialized cardiac conduction system.

coordinated contraction of the ventricles. There is a small, but important, difference in the *sequence of activation* of various portions of the ventricles, which will be discussed later.

Muscle Mass of Cardiac Chambers

The *atria* pump blood over only very short distances (across the AV valves into the ventricles); therefore, they are very thin-walled structures with very little muscle mass. Conversely, the right ventricle must pump blood all the way through the lungs, and therefore has a thicker wall and more muscle mass. Finally, the left ventricle pumps blood out to the entire body, and thus has the thickest wall of all the chambers, three to four times thicker than the wall of the right ventricle (Figure 1.3).

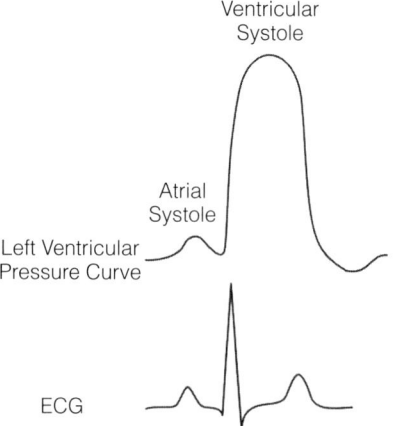

Figure 1.2. Synchronous recording of left ventricular pressure curve and ECG. The time required for mechanical contraction during atrial and ventricular systole is shown by the left ventricular pressure curve. Note how these times exceed the times required for atrial and ventricular depolarization (P wave and QRS duration.)

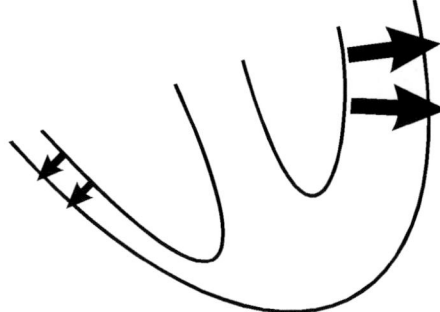

Figure 1.3. Schematic drawing showing relative greater thickness of the septum and wall of the left ventricle as compared to the right ventricle. Arrows represent force vectors, illustrating that as a result of its greater thickness, the left ventricle generates greater voltages.

One determinant of the size of an electrical complex on the electrocardiogram is how much *voltage* is generated by depolarization of a given portion of the heart. Thus, the QRS complex is normally larger than the P wave because depolarization of the greater muscle mass of the ventricles generates more voltage than does depolarization of the thinner walls of the atria.

Recording a Wave of Depolarization

A wave of depolarization spreading across a strip of muscle can be recorded by a *galvanometer*, which is an instrument that measures voltage. Figure 1.4 illustrates an isolated strip of muscle that is stimulated at the left end, producing a wave of depolarization that spreads from left to right. Three electrodes placed on this muscle strip are connected to a galvanometer. The

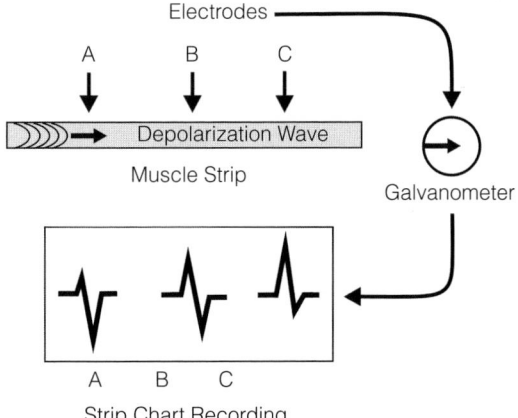

Figure 1.4. Strip chart recording of depolarization of an isolated muscle strip "viewed" by three exploring electrodes. As the wave of depolarization comes toward each electrode it produces a positive deflection on the recording. As the wave passes under the electrode the needle begins to swing down toward neutral, then inscribes a clearly negative deflection as the wave begins to move away from the electrode.

needle of the galvanometer swings up or down as the electrical events in the muscle strip are measured. These events can then be permanently recorded by attaching a pen to the end of the needle and passing a paper strip at a constant speed beneath the pen. The result is called a *strip chart recording*.

By convention, the needle swings up when an impulse is coming toward a measuring electrode and down when an impulse is going away from an electrode. Note that as the wave of depolarization in Figure 1.4 comes toward each electrode, there is an initial positive deflection seen on the corresponding recording of the strip chart. As the wave passes directly beneath each electrode, for an instant the wave is going neither toward nor away from the electrode; therefore, the needle rapidly swings down toward the neutral position. However, the wave doesn't really stop, but continues to move, immediately passing the electrode, and going away from it. This causes the needle to continue downward past the neutral position to record a negative deflection. When the wave finally reaches the end of the muscle strip and depolarization is over, the needle again swings up to the neutral position and comes to rest on what is called the *isoelectric line*.

Note that in Figure 1.4 the strip chart recordings for A, B, and C all look slightly different, depending on the position from which their electrodes "viewed" the spreading wave of depolarization. Because the wave of depolarization was spreading toward electrode C for most of the time, the corresponding C recording is predominantly upright, with only a brief negative deflection at the end. Conversely, because the impulse was spreading away from electrode A for most of the time, the strip chart recording A is predominantly negative, with only a brief initial period of positive deflection, corresponding to the short time the impulse was coming toward electrode A. This simple concept of measuring voltages in muscle from different locations or "viewpoints" is the essence of 12-lead electrocardiography.

2

Electrocardiographic Waveforms

What I called strip chart recordings A, B, and C in the first chapter, we will now refer to in ECG jargon as waveforms or complexes. This chapter will review the electrical events in the heart that correspond to each complex, the normal parameters for these complexes and the intervals between them, and finally, waveform terminology.

The ECG Grid

The familiar ECG grid consists of 1-mm squares (Figure 2.1). As you know from your previous exposure to dysrhythmias, time is measured on the horizontal axis of the grid. Each small box, which measures 1 mm horizontally, equals 0.04 s in time. The width of ECG complexes is commonly referred to as the *duration*.

You may also remember that the vertical axis is a relative measure of voltage, but is usually expressed in millimeters of positive or negative deflection, rather than in volts. The height or depth of deflection is commonly referred to as the *amplitude*.

The P Wave

The *P wave*, of course, corresponds to the depolarization of atrial muscle. Because there is relatively little atrial muscle mass, only low voltages are normally produced. The amplitude of the P wave should normally not exceed 2 or 3 mm, and its duration should not be greater than 0.11 s. Greater amplitude or duration may often indicate *enlargement* of the atria, with more than the usual amount of muscle mass (Figure 2.2).

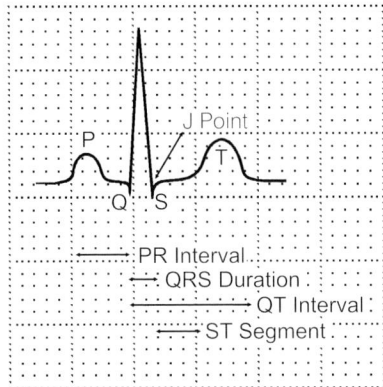

Figure 2.1. The ECG grid with waveforms and intervals. Each small box in the grid represents 0.04 s in time horizontally. The vertical axis measures relative voltage, but is usually expressed in mm of amplitude.

The PR Interval

The *PR interval* corresponds to the time it takes an impulse to travel from the SA node all the way down through the conduction system to the first muscle fibers stimulated in the ventricles. Therefore, it is measured from the beginning of the P wave to the beginning of the QRS. Note that in Figure 2.1, although you can see depolarization of the atria in the form of the P wave, you cannot see the impulse traveling through the AV node, bundle of His,

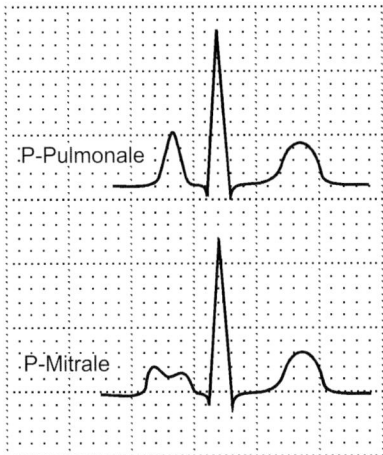

Figure 2.2. Two different kinds of P wave abnormalities seen in lead II. P-pulmonale, with tall peaked P waves, is commonly seen in patients with right atrial enlargement secondary to pulmonary hypertension. P-mitrale, which is characterized by broad, notched P waves, is commonly seen in left atrial enlargement secondary to mitral valve disease.

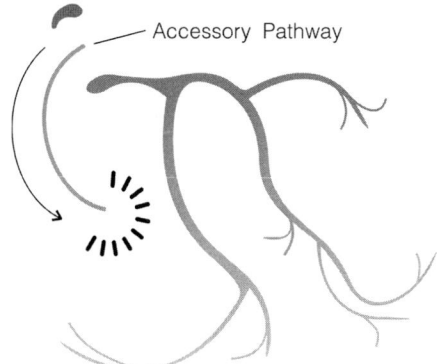
— Accessory Pathway

Figure 2.3. Schematic diagram of the specialized conduction system of the heart showing a congenital accessory pathway from atria to ventricles. The accessory pathway bypasses the AV node and rapidly conducts the impulse directly to the ventricles, producing early depolarization, or preexcitation.

bundle branches, or Purkinje fibers because the voltages in these structures are too low to register on our galvanometer.

As you will remember from your study of dysrhythmias, the normal PR interval runs from ~0.12 to 0.20 s. Shorter intervals indicate *accelerated conduction* from the atria to the ventricles, such as in *Wolf–Parkinson–White (WPW) syndrome* or in a junctional pacemaker, which you are already familiar with from your study of dysrhythmias. In WPW syndrome there are congenitally aberrant pathways (Figure 2.3) outside of the normal conduction system that bypass the slowing effect of the AV node and rapidly conduct impulses from the atria directly to the ventricles—a kind of electrical "short circuit" manifested by the classic *delta wave* (Figure 2.4).

PR intervals that are longer than 0.20 s indicate a delay in normal conduction somewhere in the conduction system between the AV node and the bifurcation of the bundle of His—the familiar *first-degree AV block*.

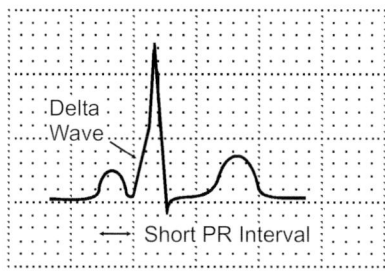
Delta Wave

Short PR Interval

Figure 2.4. Wolff-Parkinson-White syndrome as seen in lead II. Note that the ventricles are activated very early, as indicated by the delta wave beginning very shortly after the P wave. Thus, the hallmark of WPW is a delta wave, creating a very short PR interval.

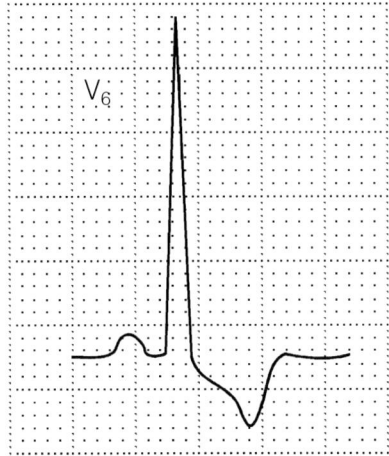

Figure 2.5. Left ventricular hypertrophy as seen in lead V_6. Note that the amplitude of the R wave exceeds 25 mm. The ST segment and T wave show a typical "strain pattern" of LVH.

The QRS

The QRS is naturally the largest complex on the ECG because it corresponds to depolarization of the ventricles, with their larger muscle mass. Therefore, QRS amplitude may normally reach as high as 25 mm or more (five big boxes) in large individuals, or in those with thin chest walls that actually allow the precordial electrodes to be closer to the heart. Amplitudes >25 mm are frequently associated with *chamber enlargement* (ventricular hypertrophy), as seen in Figure 2.5. Conversely, very low QRS amplitudes are also abnormal and may be seen with diffuse, severe cardiac disease or illnesses such as pericardial effusion and hypothyroidism.

If the conduction system is working properly, the duration of the QRS should be <0.10 s. Durations of 0.10 s or greater indicate a delay in the spread of depolarization through the ventricles, the so-called *intraventricular conduction delay*, as is seen in BBBs (Figure 2.6). More on that later.

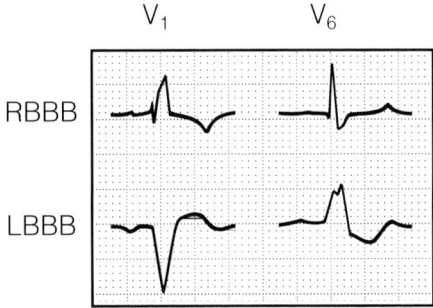

Figure 2.6. Two examples of BBB. Note that the QRS duration is increased to 0.12 s or greater, and that there is deformity of the ST and T waves, with T waves usually inscribed in the opposite direction from the QRS. The characteristic RSR′ pattern is seen in V_1 or V_2 in RBBB, and in V_5 or V_6 in LBBB.

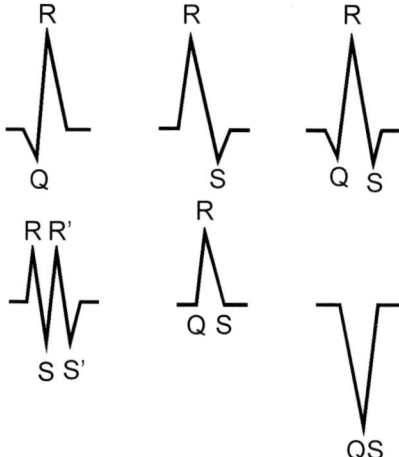

Figure 2.7. QRS Nomenclature. Note that when the complex has no Q or S wave, it is still permissible to call it a "QRS."

Later, you will see that it becomes very important to be able to describe the various combinations of positive and negative deflections of the QRS very accurately. Therefore, it is worthwhile to spend a little time now reviewing nomenclature of the QRS.

Figure 2.7 shows some of the various possible QRS inscription combinations. The rules are as follows:

1. The first deflection of the complex is called a *Q wave* if it is negative.
2. The first positive deflection of the complex is called an *R wave*.
3. A negative deflection coming after an R wave is called an *S wave*.
4. Positive deflections coming after the first R wave are labeled *R′* (*R prime*).
5. Negative deflections coming after the first S wave are labeled *S′* (*S prime*).

ST Segment

The *ST segment* represents the time between the completion of depolarization of the ventricles and the onset of repolarization of the ventricles. It is normally isoelectric, meaning neither positive nor negative, and gently blends into the upslope of the subsequent T wave (Figure 2.1). The point at which the ST segment takes off from the QRS is called the *J point*.

The ST segment plays a very important role in the diagnosis of ischemic heart disease, particularly in acute myocardial infarction (AMI). Most of you are aware that dramatic *ST segment elevation* is one of the hallmarks of AMI (Figure 2.8). Sometimes however, the ST segment may be slightly elevated above the baseline across the entire tracing in perfectly healthy people, particularly young males. This finding is called *benign early repolarization changes* and reflects a phase of repolarization of the ventricles that occurs earlier in the cardiac cycle than in most people.

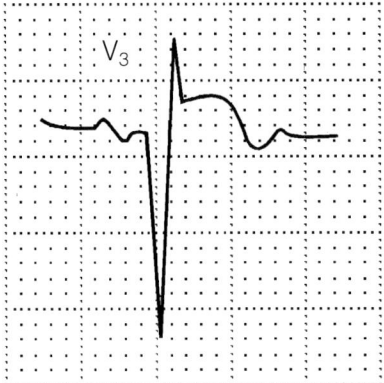

Figure 2.8. The three hallmarks of acute myocardial infarction, including ST segment elevation, T wave inversion, and Q wave formation.

The ST segment can also be *depressed* below the base line in a variety of conditions, such as ischemia and ventricular hypertrophy. ST-segment shifts of all sorts will be discussed in detail in later chapters.

The T Wave

The T wave corresponds to repolarization of the ventricles. It is normally inscribed in the same direction as the predominant deflection of the QRS, and has less amplitude than the QRS. Abnormalities of the T wave predominantly take the form of *inversion* (being inscribed in the opposite direction of the QRS), as we have seen in BBB, left ventricular hypertrophy (LVH), and AMI. They may also take the form of very large or small amplitudes, such as in hyperkalemia and hypokalemia (Figure 2.9).

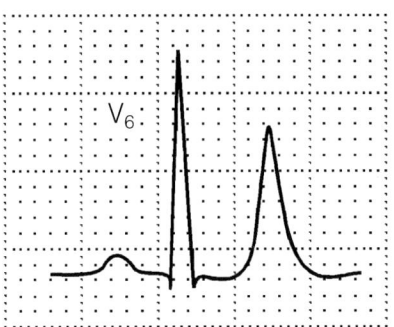

Figure 2.9. Extremely tall, pointed T waves seen with hyperkalemia.

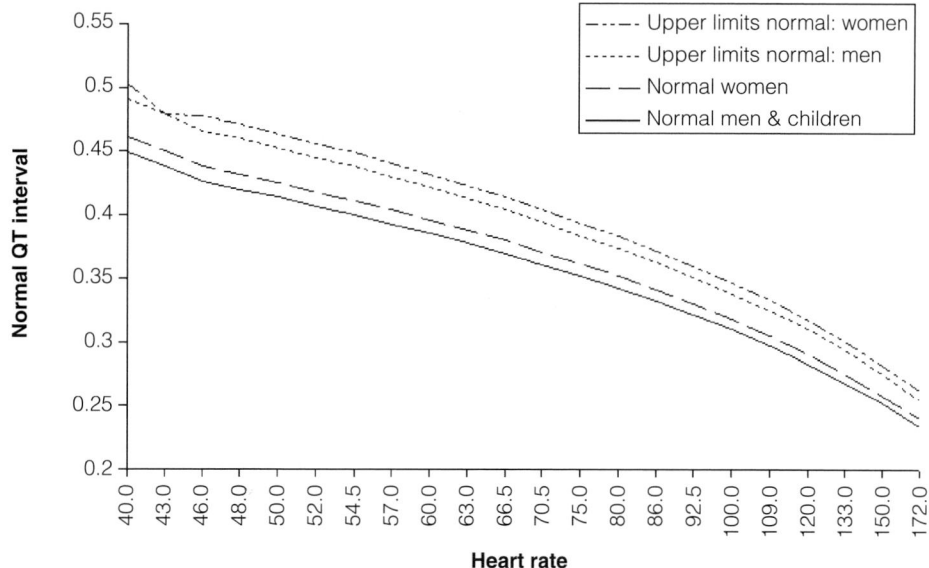

Figure 2.10. Graph plotting normal QT interval against heart rate for men, women, and children.

The QT Interval

The *QT interval* is measured from the beginning of the QRS to the end of the T wave, and normal intervals vary with heart rate and the person's sex. Therefore, when determining whether a QT interval is normal or not, it is best to use a chart that plots normal intervals against heart rate (Figure 2.10) and sex.

The primary potential abnormality of the QT interval is *prolongation*, reflecting delays in ventricular repolarization. This is commonly the result of the administration of drugs, such as procainamide or quinidine, or of electrolyte imbalance, particularly as in hypocalcemia. When the QT interval is prolonged, there is a greater opportunity for R-on-T phenomenon, and a higher incidence of ventricular reentry dysrhythmias and sudden death.

A Word About Nonspecific ST and T Wave Changes

Frequent readers of electrocardiogram reports will be frustratingly familiar with the term *nonspecific ST and T wave changes*. This term reflects the unfortunate reality that the electrocardiogram has significant limitations as a diagnostic tool, and that there are many ECG abnormalities that have more than one cause and are therefore not specific for any one disease state. Thus, the term nonspecific has a genuine usefulness in calling the reader's attention to waveform changes that are abnormal, but cannot be ascribed to any single cause.

3

Cardiac Vectors and Lead Systems

In Chapter 3, I will discuss the concept of vectors, the sequences of activation of heart muscle, and the directions from which various leads "look" at the heart. All setting the stage for figuring out what the normal ECG looks like in each lead and why.

Force Vectors

Undoubtedly, you have heard it said that wavefronts of depolarization do not really travel in straight lines, but spread over tissue like a ripple in a pond spreads out from the point where you toss a stone. This is actually a quite good analogy, but is difficult to illustrate in a diagram. It has always been easier to describe the direction in which a wave is traveling and the magnitude of its force (in this case voltage) by using arrows.

Thus, in Figure 3.1, we see an attempt to depict a wavefront of depolarization (spreading from endocardium to epicardium) with curved lines, representing the spreading edge of the wavefront, and short arrows, representing both the direction in which the wavefront is traveling and its relative force (voltage). These arrows are called *force vectors*.

If we mentally eliminate the curved lines and keep just the arrows to represent the wavefront, we can easily see that the sum of all the little arrows can be represented by the one larger arrow in the middle of the diagram. This larger arrow represents the *mean* direction of the wavefront and its relative force. It is called a *summation vector* because it represents the sum of all the little vectors. The larger the arrow, the greater the force.

Sequences of Depolarization

It is possible to simply illustrate the major sequences of depolarization of the heart and the relative voltages encountered by drawing a series of summation vectors (Figure 3.2). It is also useful to describe the direction in which these vectors are traveling by superimposing our drawing on a 360-degree compass rose. We will modify our standard compass rose a little bit, however,

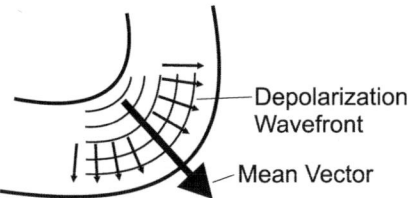

Figure 3.1. Schematic section through a ventricle shows the spread of a wave of depolarization from endocardium to epicardium. The wavefront and its relative force is shown by the series of small arrows. The mean direction of the wavefront and its mean force are represented by the large arrow.

by assigning the zero-degree mark to the horizontal on the right and going clockwise with positive degrees to +180 degree and counterclockwise with negative degrees to −180 degree. This is done by *convention* (by general agreement) in electrocardiography.

Note in Figure 3.2 that vector 1 represents depolarization of the atria and that the wavefront spreads down over the atria toward the patient's left at roughly a 40- to 50-degree angle. This vector would obviously correspond to the P wave of the ECG.

Vector 2 represents depolarization of the ventricular septum, the first part of the ventricles to be activated, and corresponds to the first deflection of the QRS complex. Note that depolarization of the septum normally takes place from left to right. This is because the impulse normally travels somewhat faster down the left bundle branch than down the right bundle branch. Therefore, the left side of the septum is activated first.

Vector 3 represents the summation vector of depolarization of the bulk of ventricular muscle and therefore corresponds to the *main deflection* of the QRS. Note that this vector is normally angled slightly to the left, at approximately 60 degrees, despite the fact that depolarization of both ventricles is

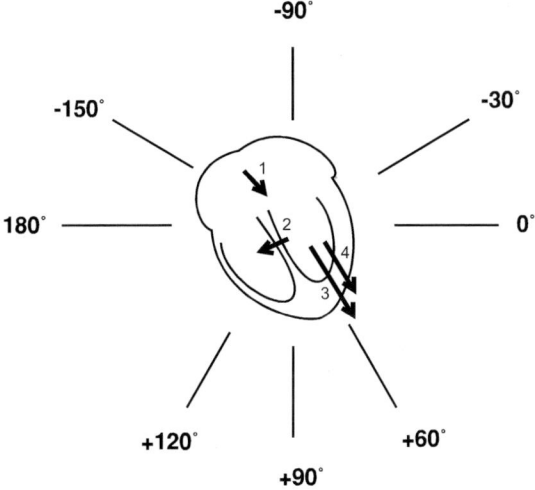

Figure 3.2. Summation vectors of cardiac depolarization.

initiated almost simultaneously. This is so for three reasons. First, the considerably greater muscle mass of the left ventricle generates greater voltages than does the right ventricle, with the result that the summation vector is shifted leftward. Second, it takes more time for the wavefront to pass through the wall of the left ventricle than that of the right ventricle because of the considerably greater thickness of the left ventricular wall. This leaves the electrical forces in the left ventricle relatively unopposed during the later part of ventricular depolarization, and thus, also serves to shift the summation vector leftward. Finally, the position of the heart itself in the chest cavity is such that the apex is tilted slightly toward the left, as seen in Figure 3.2.

Vector 4 is the resultant of the electrical forces generated by repolarization of the ventricles and therefore is responsible for producing the T wave of the ECG. Because repolarization is a slower process than depolarization, the T wave does not have the same sharp configuration as the QRS. Vector 4 is generally inclined at approximately the same angle as the main vector of ventricular depolarization. Therefore, the inscription of the T wave on the ECG is usually in the same direction as the major deflection of the QRS.

Lead Systems

The exact placement of the leads in the standard 12-lead ECG is the result of general agreement that has evolved over the years among electrocardiographers. Many additional lead locations other than the usual are possible. We will avoid, however, a discussion of the actual physical placement of leads and the theory of Einthoven's Triangle because it is not necessary to your understanding of ECG morphology and frequently results in confusion. Suffice it to say that the simpler description of lead systems that follows is entirely sufficient to support an accurate interpretation of the ECG.

We saw in Chapter 1 that the strip chart recordings of electrical events in a strip of muscle look different, depending on the position of the electrode that views the events. The 12 leads of the standard 12-lead ECG were selected to offer a wide variety of "views" of the heart.

Although a technical oversimplification, the following description of the leads in the 12-lead ECG is a useful, and clinically quite accurate, method of conceptualizing lead systems.

The 12-lead ECG "looks" at the heart in two different planes (Figure 3.3). The three so-called *standard limb leads* (I, II, and III), and the three so-called *augmented limb leads* (aVR, aVL, and aVF) all look at the heart from the "edges" of the *frontal plane*, as if the body was flat or unidimensional. It is common practice to refer to all six leads, collectively, simply as the *limb leads*.

The six *V leads* (V_1-V_6) across the precordium look at the heart in the horizontal or *transverse* plane (Figure 3.3). These leads allow us to look at the front and left side of the heart and complete a more three-dimensional perspective.

Note in Figure 3.4 that to describe from which direction each of the limb leads looks at the heart in the frontal plane, we have again used our modified compass rose. It is useful to think of each lead as being an *exploring elec-*

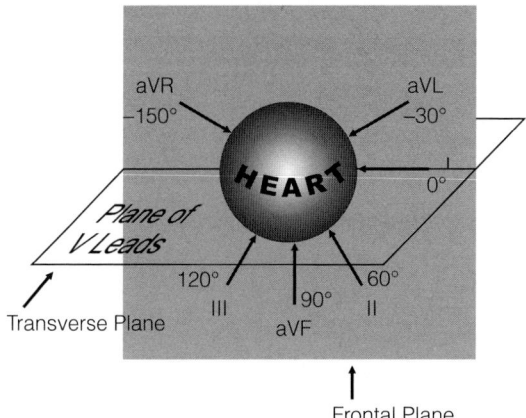

Figure 3.3. The 12-lead electrocardiogram "looks" at the heart in two different planes. The limb leads examine the heart in the frontal plane, while the V leads examine the heart in the transverse plane.

trode (an electrode that explores the heart) located in the positions shown in the figure. In actuality, of course, this is not the case. Rather, the ECG machine manipulates signals in its internal circuitry to give us tracings that look much as if electrodes were placed in those positions.

One can readily see then that aVR "looks down" on the heart from above and to the right, at a position of −150 degrees. Lead aVL looks down on the heart from above and to the left, at −30 degrees. Lead I looks at the heart on the horizontal, directly from the left side, at 0 degrees. Finally, leads II, aVF, and III all look "up" at the heart from below and, together, are called the *inferior leads* because they look at the inferior wall of the heart from the angles shown in Figure 3.4. By the same token, leads I and aVL are said to look at the *lateral* and *high lateral* walls of the heart, respectively.

This system of superimposing each of the limb leads on our modified compass rose is called the *hexaxial reference system*. You are urged to

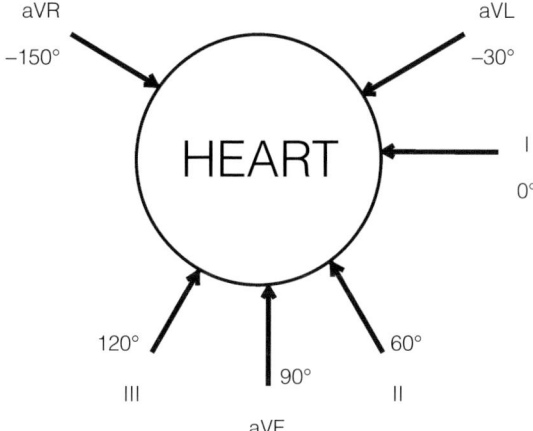

Figure 3.4. The hexaxial reference system showing the direction from which each of the limb leads "looks" at the heart in the frontal plane.

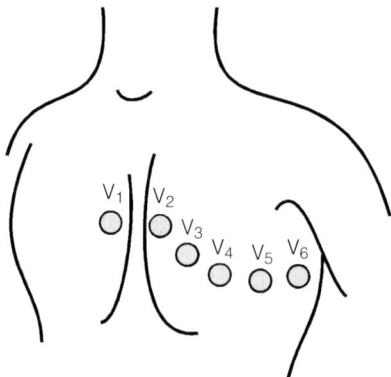

Figure 3.5. Position of the six V leads across the precordium.

memorize these positions and their assigned degree values because the hexaxial reference system will become your primary tool later on when you learn to determine the electrical axis of the heart.

In the same manner as the limb leads, the V leads, across the precordium of the chest, "look" at the heart in the transverse plane from the positions shown in Figure 3.5. In the case of the V leads, however, we do not use degrees on a compass rose to assign positions. Rather positions are assigned on the basis of actual location of the exploring electrodes as follows:

V_1—right sternal border, 4th interspace
V_2—left sternal border, 4th interspace
V_3—midway between V_2 and V_4
V_4—midclavicular line, 5th interspace
V_5—anterior axillary line, 5th interspace
V_6—midaxillary line, 5th interspace

You will learn in later chapters that, particularly in diagnosing AMI, small changes in the height of the R wave on the V-lead recordings across the precordium can be important. Artifactual changes in R-wave height can be produced merely by slightly moving the positions of the V electrodes. Therefore, it is important when following serial ECG tracings to make certain that the V leads are placed in exactly the same position each time an ECG is performed. To this end, it is a good idea to mark the positions on the chest wall with indelible ink pen at the time of the first tracing so that subsequent tracings can be done with the V leads in exactly the same positions.

4

Derivation of the Normal Electrocardiogram

One of the most intimidating aspects of 12-lead ECG, preventing many students from pursuing that discipline, is the thought that one will never be able to memorize what the normal ECG looks like in all those different leads. Without realizing it, however, you have now acquired all the skills necessary to predict what the ECG will look like in each lead. Rather than memorizing, in this chapter we will figure it out together.

Important Principles

Knowledge of the following three concepts (with which you are already acquainted) is almost all that is necessary to predict the normal *morphology*, or shape, of the ECG tracing in each lead:

1. The principle that impulses coming toward an electrode produce positive deflections, whereas impulses going away from an electrode produce negative deflections.
2. The positions from which the various electrodes "look" at the heart.
3. The sequence, direction, and relative magnitude of the four major vectors of cardiac depolarization and repolarization.

There is just one more principle of which you need to be aware, which is only a slight amplification of principle number 1. Figure 4.1 illustrates the principle that the more directly an impulse comes toward an electrode, the greater the amplitude of the positive recorded deflection will be. Vector A in the illustration is coming directly toward the recording electrode and produces a very tall deflection in recording A. Vector B, on the other hand, is not coming as directly toward the electrode, and therefore produces a deflection of less magnitude in recording B; that is, the positive deflection is shorter.

The same is true of impulses going away from an electrode, only the deflections are negative instead of positive. The more directly an impulse goes away from an electrode, the deeper will be the negative deflection, and the less directly an impulse goes away from an electrode, the shallower will be the negative deflection. Vector C is going directly away from the electrode, and so produces a deep negative deflection. Vector D, on the other hand, is not going as directly away and so produces a deflection of lesser amplitude; that is, the deflection is shallower.

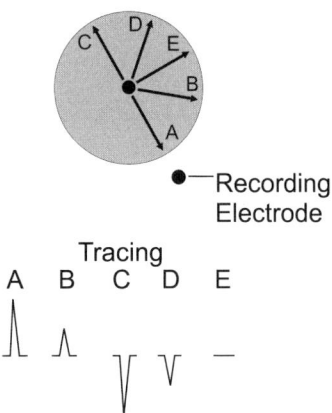

Figure 4.1. Diagram of five force vectors of equal magnitude, but different directions, as recorded by a single exploring electrode.

Finally, when an impulse is traveling exactly perpendicular to an electrode, that is, when it is neither coming toward nor going away from the electrode, the recorded deflection will be either isoelectric or *biphasic*, with positive and negative deflections of equal amplitude. Vector E illustrates this result.

The Normal Electrocardiogram

Now we have all the tools we need to begin to predict the normal ECG tracing in each lead. To help us, we will superimpose our drawing of the major vectors of cardiac depolarization on top of the hexaxial reference system as seen in Figure 4.2.

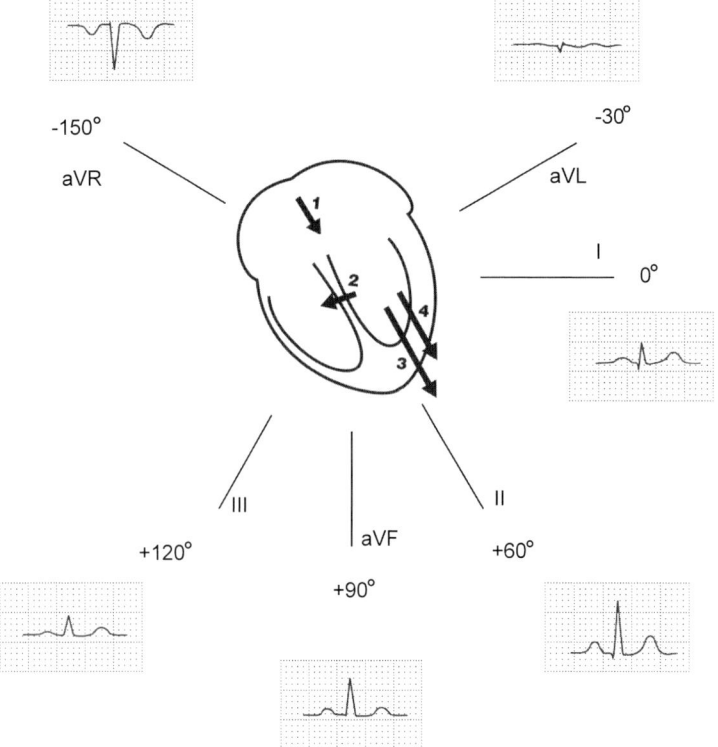

Figure 4.2. Derivation of the normal electrocardiogram in the six limb leads.

Lead II

Let's begin with limb lead II. Lead II is located below the heart and to the left at 60 degrees. Vector 1 represents depolarization of the atria and is coming almost directly at lead II. Because it is coming directly at lead II, we would expect a positive P wave that is quite tall and, actually, should be taller than in any other lead. That, in fact, is the case. Now you know why for so many years lead II has been used as one of the primary monitoring leads; it normally has the tallest P waves, and as a result, it is one of the leads in which it is easiest to diagnose dysrhythmias.

Vector 2 represents depolarization of the ventricular septum, so it will produce the first deflection of our QRS. It is a relatively small vector without a great deal of force. In addition, it is almost perpendicular to lead II, but is, perhaps, going slightly more away from than toward lead II. So we might expect, at most, a tiny negative deflection of low amplitude as the first deflection of our QRS in lead II. Indeed, we see in our tracing that lead II usually has a very small Q wave.

Next comes Vector 3, the large summation vector of main ventricular depolarization. It is coming virtually head-on toward lead II, so we will expect that the main deflection of our QRS will be positive and quite tall. And, of course, we see in our tracing that lead II has the tallest R wave of all the limb leads because Vector 3 is coming more directly at lead II than at any other lead.

Finally, Vector 4, representing the T wave, is also coming just about directly toward lead II, so we would expect the T wave in lead II also to be positive, and probably also to be the tallest of any of the limb lead T waves. Again we see in our tracings that this is, in fact, the case.

Lead aVR

Next, let's examine aVR because it nicely illustrates what happens when vectors are going away from a lead. Remember that aVR looks down on the heart from above and to the right at −150 degrees.

Vector 1, our P wave vector, is going almost directly away from lead aVR, so we will expect our P wave to be negative and quite deep.

Vector 2, the vector of our first QRS deflection, is actually coming slightly more toward than away from lead aVR. So perhaps the first deflection of our QRS will be positive, but if so, it certainly should be of very low amplitude, and indeed, in Figure 4.2 we do see a tiny R wave in lead aVR as a quite normal finding.

One can easily see, however, that a very slight counterclockwise shift in the direction of vector 2 would mean that it was going more away from aVR than toward it, in which case we would no longer have a small R wave. The same shift in direction, rotating the vector more toward lead II, would cause us to lose our small Q wave in lead II. Indeed, it is for this reason that the presence of both the small R wave in aVR and the small Q wave in lead II are normally variable.

Vector 3, our vector of main QRS deflection, is, like the P wave vector, going almost, but not quite, directly away from lead aVR. So we expect a predominantly negative S wave in aVR, but it should not be quite as deep as the lead II R wave is tall. This is because Vector 3 is going directly toward lead II, although not as directly away from aVR. The QRS in lead aVR will therefore not register quite as much voltage as will the QRS in lead II.

Similarly, we can expect vector 4 to produce a negative T wave in aVR, again, of slightly lesser amplitude than the positive T wave in lead II.

Lead aVL

Lead aVL is the lead that is normally the most perpendicular to Vector 3, which is the vector of main ventricular depolarization. If the direction of vector 3 is +60 degrees and aVL is looking at the vector from −30 degrees, then aVL is at exactly a right angle (90 degrees) to vector 3.

Because our P wave vector is inclined at slightly less than +60 degrees, it is going more toward than away from aVL, and our P wave should therefore be positive, but of low amplitude.

Vector 2 is clearly traveling away from aVL, so a readily visible Q wave in aVL is not surprising.

Vector 3, at +60 degrees, is exactly perpendicular to aVL, so we would expect our QRS to be equally biphasic and of low amplitude.

Vector 4, which is also at right angles to aVL, may produce a practically isoelectric T wave.

Note that very minor changes, in either direction, of Vectors 1, 3, or 4 could make the ECG tracing in lead AVL either predominantly positive or predominantly negative. For this reason, the P, QRS, and T waves may be normally either positive or negative in lead aVL, although they all commonly follow each other in the direction of inscription.

Lead III

Vector 1 will clearly produce a positive P wave in Lead III, although not as tall as the P wave we saw in Lead II.

In the case of vector 2, we now have a situation in which the direction of septal depolarization is coming toward our electrode. As a result, a small positive deflection is produced, which simply contributes to the height of the R wave rather than producing a small Q wave as we saw in Leads aVL and II.

Vector 3, of course, produces a predominantly positive QRS, but, again, the R wave is not as tall as in lead II because Vector 3 is coming less directly toward lead III. As usual, the T wave simply follows the predominant direction of the QRS.

Leads I and aVF

The reader can now go through the same exercise with the two remaining leads (I and aVF) and easily derive the normal ECG pattern in each one. It is obvious that lead I will have a pattern somewhat intermediate between that of aVL and II and that lead aVF will have a pattern that falls between the patterns of leads II and III.

The V Leads

We can now go through a similar exercise in predicting what the normal V leads will look like. Figure 4.3 shows the position of the precordial electrodes in relation to the heart. It is important to understand that the exact position of the electrodes in relation to the heart varies from person to person, as well as from technician to technician.

The V_1 electrode may be slightly to the right of (above) the atria, over the mid–right atrium, or even to the left of (below) the atrium, but it is always above the ventricles. For this reason, the P waves in V_1 of the normal ECG may be negative, biphasic, or positive, but the QRS is always negative (Figure 4.4).

In most people, V_1 actually looks very much like aVR because the main vector of ventricular depolarization is going away from both leads.

As in aVR, there is a small R wave in V_1, reflecting septal depolarization. By the same token, septal depolarization is also responsible for producing a small normal Q wave in the left precordial leads, V_5 and V_6.

Somewhere in the vicinity of V_2 to V_4, the electrode usually reaches the level of the midventricle. At this point, the P waves are naturally positive, and the QRS becomes biphasic because the electrode is beginning to pick up the small vectors coming toward it from endocardium to epicardium over the right ventricle, as well as the vectors spreading away from it down over the left ventricle. Note in Figure 4.3 that the left ventricle actually lies posterior to the right ventricle.

The point at which the QRS becomes biphasic is called the *transition zone* because it is here that the predominant QRS deflection transitions from negative to positive. One of the results of this transition is that the R wave, normally small in V_1, progressively increases in height as one moves from right to left across the precordium, until the QRS is fully upright in leads V_5 and

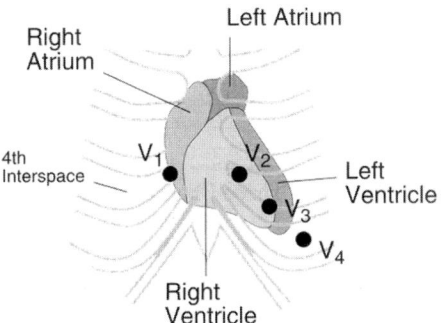

Figure 4.3. Position of the V leads. Diagram illustrating the position of the V leads relative to the heart anteriorly. V_5 and V_6 are positioned in the same interspace as V_4 (the 5th interspace), but go into the page laterally around the patient's left side. Note that the right ventricle actually lies anterior to the left ventricle, as well as to the right, and that the apex of the heart is pointed slightly to the left.

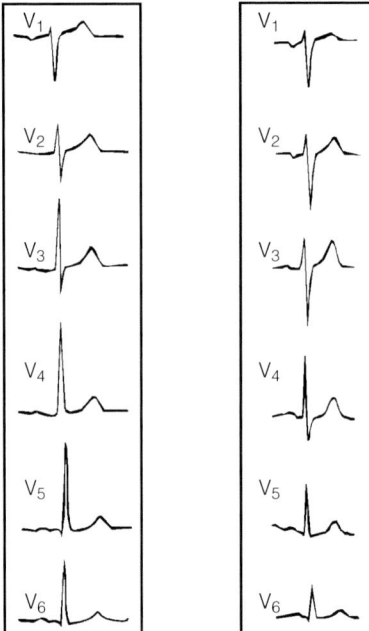

Figure 4.4. The normal V leads. The first tracing displays a transition zone in V_2; the second in leads V_3 and V_4.

V_6. You will later learn that this normal *R wave progression* is frequently lost in anterior wall myocardial infarction.

The T wave is variable in leads V_1 and V_2, but normally becomes upright by the time one reaches the transition zone.

In summary, anything can happen with regard to P waves and T waves in V_1 and V_2, but they should both be upright by lead V_3. The QRS should always be predominantly negative in V_1, can be biphasic from leads V_2 to V_4, and should always be upright in leads V_5 and V_6.

The Layout of Three-Channel Tracings

Now that we have deduced the normal morphology of the electrocardiogram in each individual lead, we can finally put them all together in a full, normal 12-lead ECG as seen in Figure 4.5. This ECG tracing shows the usual order of lead display utilized by today's three-channel machines. All three horizontal panels are displaying the same beats, simultaneously seen in three leads. The opportunity to see each beat in three leads simultaneously is especially helpful in the diagnosis of dysrhythmias.

Note that as the machine changes leads in each of the three panels, there is no pause at the time of lead change, so calipers can be used to plot intervals all the way across the tracing without interruption.

Also note that in this example (Figure 4.5) of a normal ECG, lead III is almost equally biphasic and lead I has a slightly more positive deflection than

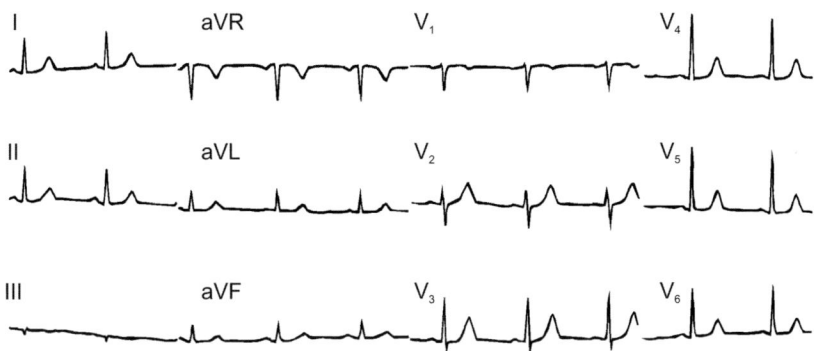

Figure 4.5. A normal 12-lead electrocardiogram. Note that in this example, both the P wave and the T wave are inverted in V_1. The transition zone occurs in V_2.

in Figure 4.2. This means that, in this quite normal patient, all of our vectors (vectors 1 to 4) are inclined slightly more counterclockwise (to the patient's left) than in Figure 4.2. Because lead III is almost isoelectric, vector 3 must be at approximately a right angle to lead III, or at approximately 30 degrees. Without realizing it, you have just determined the electrical axis of this tracing, which is the subject of our next chapter.

5

Electrical Axis

In Chapter 5, you will discover, happily enough, that you also now have all the tools necessary to determine electrical axis, a fairly easy exercise that has the unfair reputation of being difficult.

The Definition of Electrical Axis

The term *electrical axis* normally refers to nothing more than determining the direction, or angle in degrees, in which is pointed the main vector of ventricular depolarization; that is, the direction of our old friend, vector 3. For the purpose of determining electrical axis, we therefore use the by now familiar hexaxial reference system. The precordial V leads are not used in the determination of electrical axis.

We said earlier that, in the average person, vector 3 has a direction of approximately 60 degrees. Although 60 degrees is the average, there is actually a wide range of normal, as is usually the case among human beings. Most authorities agree that the main summation vector of ventricular depolarization can quite normally point anywhere between *0 and 90 degrees*.

When the vector points further counterclockwise than 0 degrees, we say that the tracing displays *left axis deviation* (LAD) because the vector is pointing off to the left (Figure 5.1). When the vector points further *clockwise* than 90 degrees, we say that the tracing displays *right axis deviation* (RAD) because the vector is pointing off to the right. If the deviation from normal is greater than −30 or +120 degrees, most electrocardiographers then call it *marked* left or *marked* RAD. Deviations of less than this are usually described as *slight*.

How to Determine Electrical Axis

The Tallest R Wave

We know from previous chapters that the limb lead with the tallest R wave is going to be the lead at which vector 3 is most directly pointed. So the easiest way to roughly determine electrical axis is simply to look for the limb lead

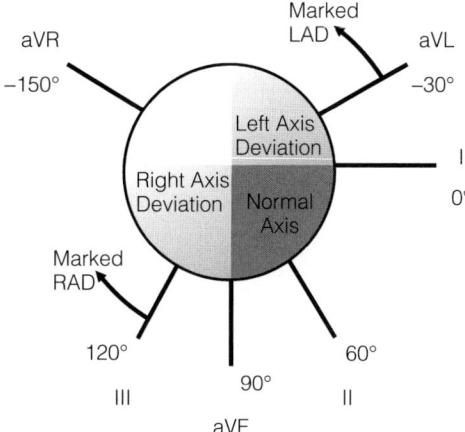

Figure 5.1. The hexaxial reference system shaded to show regions of normal axis and axis deviation.

with the tallest R wave. We then know that vector 3 is pointed roughly in that direction or at least closer to that lead than to any other lead. Thus, as is illustrated in Figure 5.2A, if the tallest R wave is seen in lead II, we know that the axis is roughly +60 degrees. If, on the other hand, the tallest R wave is seen in lead aVL, as in Figure 5.2B, we know that the axis is roughly −30 degrees, and so on.

The Deepest S Wave

It is also easy to understand, from our previous discussion of the derivation of the normal ECG, that an alternate method of roughly determining axis would be to look for the lead with the deepest negative deflection or S wave. We would then know that vector 3 was going more directly away from that lead than from any other lead. Therefore, the axis of vector 3 should be in roughly the opposite direction, or 180 degrees from the lead with the deepest S wave. If aVR has the deepest S wave, then the electrical axis should be directly opposite on the hexaxial reference system, or roughly +30 degrees (Figure 5.2C).

90 Degrees from an Equally Biphasic QRS

The aforementioned two methods of determining axis provide us with only a rough indication of the direction of the main ventricular depolarization vector. To be more accurate, we will have to refine our methods.

A third, more accurate method of determining axis is to look for a QRS that is either *equally biphasic* (that is, the positive and negative deflections are of equal amplitude) or essentially isoelectric. We know from previous discussions that when we see a lead with an equally biphasic QRS, it means that vector 3 is perpendicular to that lead.

The ECG in Figure 5.2C shows an equally biphasic QRS in lead III. So we know that our vector is perpendicular to, or 90 degrees from, this lead. What we can't tell from looking solely at lead III, however, is whether the perpendicular vector is pointed toward the right lower quadrant or the left upper quadrant of our hexaxial reference system. To determine which quadrant, we simply look for the tallest R wave, which in this case we find in lead II. Now

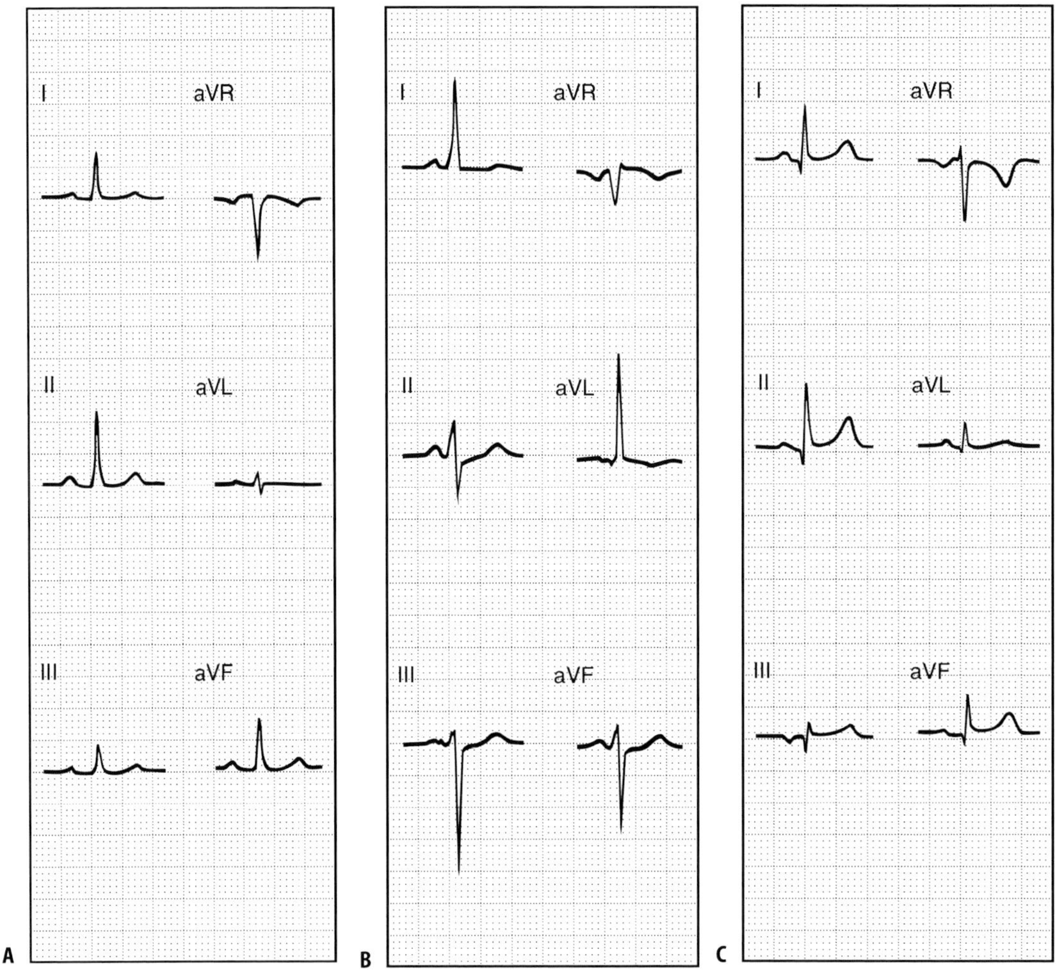

Figure 5.2 A. Patient A. The tallest R wave is seen lead II, placing the axis at approximately +60 degrees. **B.** Patient B. The tallest R wave is seen in lead aVL, placing the axis at approximately −30 degrees. **C.** Patient C. The deepest S wave is seen in lead aVR, placing the axis roughly directly opposite aVR, or at approximately 30 degrees. An equally biphasic QRS in lead III places the axis perpendicular to lead III, or also at approximately 30 degrees.

we can determine the axis to be approximately 90 degrees from lead III pointed toward the right lower quadrant, or, 30 degrees.

But what if we can't find a QRS that is exactly equally biphasic? In that instance we look for the QRS that comes closest to being equally biphasic. If it's a little more positive than negative, then we know that the vector is coming slightly more toward than away from that lead, and therefore the axis will be slightly <90 degrees from our biphasic QRS. If, on the other hand, the negative deflection is of slightly greater amplitude than the positive deflection, we know that the vector is pointed slightly more away from our lead than 90 degrees. Figure 5.2B shows a biphasic QRS in lead II that is slightly more negative than positive. Therefore, we know that the axis is actually slightly further counterclockwise from II than 90 degrees, perhaps approximately 95 degrees counterclockwise. A more refined determination would, thus, place the axis in Figure 5.2B at approximately −35 degrees.

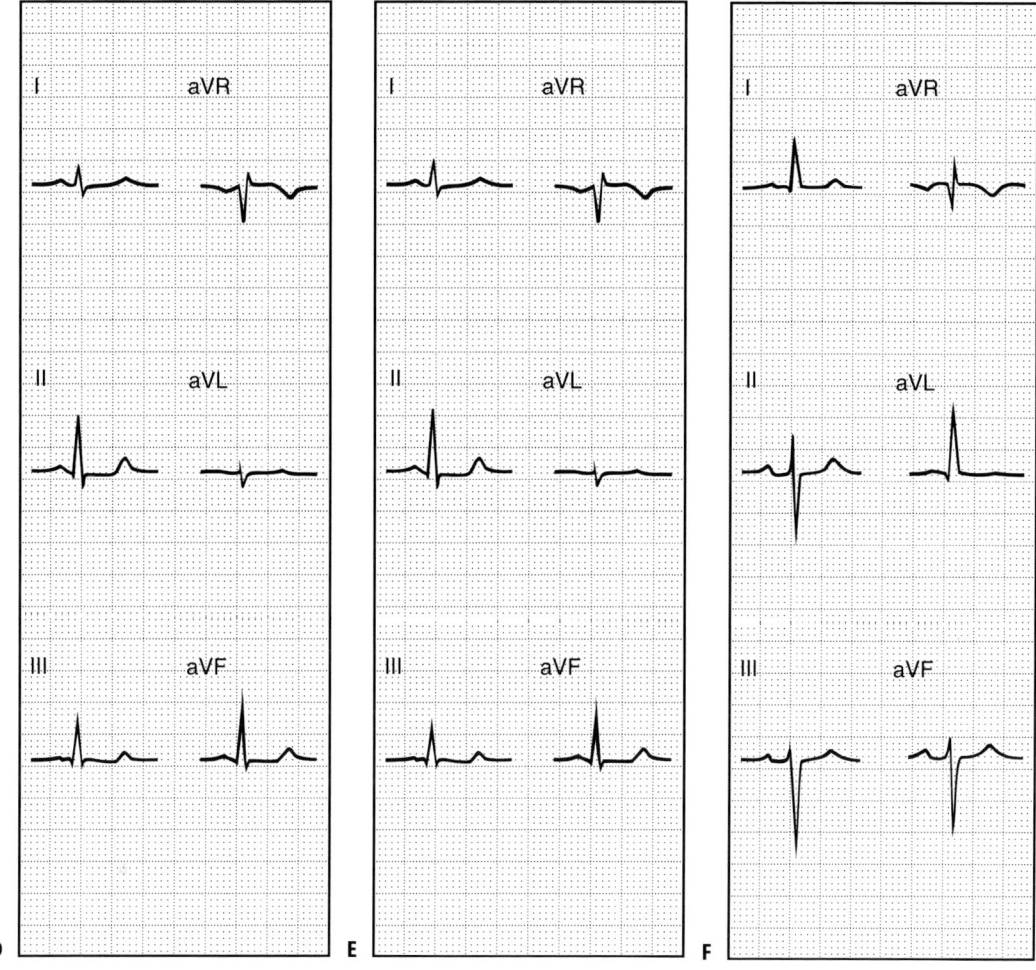

Figure 5.2 D. Patient D. Leads II and aVF are of equal amplitude, placing the axis midway between the two leads, or at 75 degrees. **E.** Patient E. Lead II has a slightly taller R wave than lead aVF, shifting the axis slightly more toward II, or approximately 70 degrees. **F.** Patient F. Lead aVR is equally biphasic, placing the axis at −60 degrees.

Midway Between the Two Equally Tallest R Waves

Obviously, not every patient is going to make it easy on us by having an electrical axis that is pointed exactly at a given lead or exactly perpendicular to a given lead. More frequently, the axis will point somewhere between two adjacent leads.

Let's say that we have a patient with an axis of 75 degrees. That would mean that our vector was pointing exactly midway between leads II and aVF. In this instance, we would expect that instead of having one lead with the tallest R wave, we would have two leads with equally tall R waves, namely II and aVF (Figure 5.2D). It is clear then that locating the axis midway between the two tallest R waves of equal height improves our accuracy.

Shifted Toward the Taller of the Two Tallest R Waves

But what if the two tallest R waves are not of equal height—what if one is slightly taller than the other? In this instance we need to shift our estimation of the axis slightly more toward the taller of the two R waves. For example, if our patient above had an axis of 70 degrees, instead of 75 degrees, then the vector would be going slightly more toward II than toward aVF, and lead II would therefore have a slightly taller R wave than aVF (Figure 5.2E).

A word of caution here. This method works only when the axis is in the right lower quadrant between 0 and 90 degrees (leads I and aVF). The reason for this can be seen by examining the tracing in Figure 5.2F. Note that lead aVL has the tallest R wave and lead I has the next tallest R wave. If we use only the method of placing the axis between the two tallest R waves and then shifting toward the taller of the two, we would estimate the axis to be approximately −20 or −25 degrees. However, if we look for an isoelectric lead, we find that lead aVR is equally biphasic. That would place the axis at −60 degrees. In this case, both leads I and aVL would be expected to be positive, with lead aVL taller than I because the vector is going more directly toward lead aVL than toward lead I; indeed, when we look at the tracing, we find that to be the case. Thus, when outside the right lower quadrant of the hexaxial reference system, we cannot reliably use alone the method of placing the axis between the two tallest R waves, and then shifting it toward the taller of the two.

Putting It All Together

After a little practice in determining axis, you will find yourself able to do it without consciously thinking about it and naturally using all of the above methods in a very rapid sequence. A very quick glance for the tallest R wave establishes the general direction of the axis. Looking for an equally biphasic QRS is usually the next natural step, followed by a quick adjustment of slightly shifting the axis based on whether the positive or negative deflection is the greater in our biphasic QRS. Finally, for axes within the right lower quadrant, we can shift the axis slightly more toward the taller of the two tallest R waves. With a little practice, you will find yourself capable of determining the axis within 10 or 15 degrees in a matter of seconds.

The Significance of Axis Deviation

Why bother determining axis in the first place? Because the term electrical axis generally refers to the direction of the vector of main ventricular depolarization, anything that changes the determinants of the direction of ventricular depolarization can cause an axis shift.

We know from previous discussions that the factors that cause the average vector of ventricular depolarization to be at 60 degrees include the sequence with which the various portions of ventricular muscle are activated and the normally greater muscle mass of the left ventricle, as well as, obviously, the physical position of the heart itself within the chest cavity. So anything that changes the sequence of ventricular activation, the muscle mass of either ventricle, or the position of the heart within the chest can cause axis deviation.

Before you go on, take a little time now to try to figure out, on the basis of this information, what disease processes might be expected to cause axis deviation. Then compare your list with the list at the end of the chapter. With a little thought, you may find that you have guessed quite a few of them, and you will learn why understanding is a much better method of learning than memorizing.

You will learn also, in later chapters, that right or LAD is a part of the criteria for many electrocardiographic diagnoses. Now, we will reveal some of the causes of axis deviation.

Sequences of Ventricular Activation

Common causes of a change in the sequence of ventricular activation that will result in axis deviation obviously include delays in conduction through either the right or left bundle branches or through one or the other of the two left hemibundles. A conduction delay or block in any one of these structures will change the sequence with which the various portions of the ventricles are activated, and thus, will change the direction of travel of the main vector of ventricular depolarization.

For example, if the right bundle branch is blocked, then the impulse will go down the left bundle normally, activating the left ventricle first. The only way for the right ventricle to then be depolarized is for the depolarization wave to spread across muscle from the left ventricle to the right ventricle. This produces a large vector spreading from left to right, and so may cause RAD (Figure 5.3).

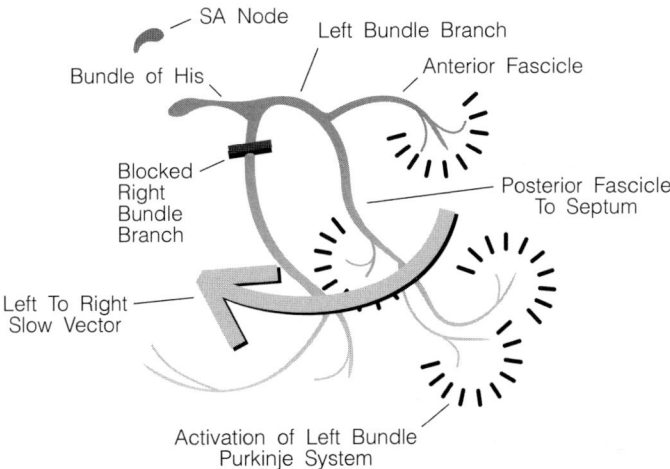

Figure 5.3. Schematic showing one of the kinds of change in sequence of activation of the ventricles that can shift electrical axis. In this example, RBBB is present. The impulse comes down the left bundle normally, activating the left ventricle via the Purkinje system. The right bundle, however, fails to conduct the impulse, and the right ventricle is depolarized by a wave of depolarization spreading across muscle from the left ventricle to the right ventricle. This may shift the main vector of ventricular depolarization to the right, producing RAD.

Changes in Ventricular Muscle Mass

You will recall that the relatively greater muscle mass of the left ventricle is one of the factors that shifted our normal vector of main ventricular depolarization slightly toward the left ventricle. This is because larger muscle masses generate greater voltages. By the same token, if we have a disease that causes right ventricular hypertrophy (RVH), such as pulmonic valve stenosis, then the enlarging muscle mass of the right ventricle will tend to shift the axis of our main vector toward the right ventricle, which may cause RAD.

Physical or Mechanical Changes in the Position of the Heart

Finally, we could obviously change the direction of our main vector of ventricular depolarization by simply altering the position of the heart within the chest cavity. A simple example is the quite healthy and normal state of pregnancy. The growing uterus puts pressure on the bottom of the diaphragm, pushing the apex of the heart up to the left into a more horizontal position, thereby mechanically altering the direction of Vector 3 and producing LAD.

Major Causes of LAD

Left BBB (LBBB)
Left anterior Hemiblock (LAH)
Premature ventricular contractions (PVCs) from the right ventricle
WPW syndrome activating the right ventricle
LVH
Pregnancy
Ascites
Abdominal tumors
Exhalation

Major Causes of RAD

Right BBB (RBBB)
Left posterior hemiblock
PVCs from the left ventricle
WPW syndrome activating the left ventricle
Emphysema
Inhalation

A Word About Indeterminate Axis

Occasionally, you will see an ECG in which all of the limb leads display an equally biphasic QRS, making determination of a single axis impossible. In such instances, you will often see the axis described as being *indeterminate* (Figure 5.4).

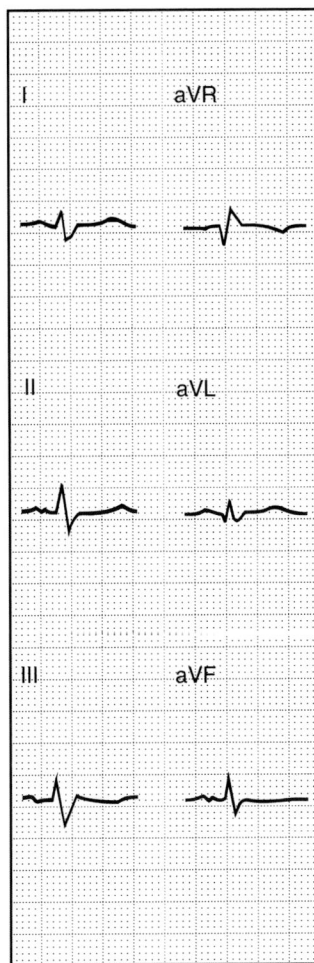

Figure 5.4. Indeterminate axis. A single axis cannot be calculated for this tracing, which shows an almost equally biphasic QRS in all leads.

Axis of P and T Waves

Although the term electrical axis, in general parlance, refers to the axis of main ventricular depolarization, it is obviously also possible to determine, in exactly the same fashion, the axis of the P wave or of the T wave. Although sometimes useful, determining the axis of these other two waves is not usually considered a routine part of ECG interpretation.

Practice Tracings

Figures 5.5–5.8 offer you some practice in your newly acquired skill of determining electrical axis. The answers may be found in Chapter 14.

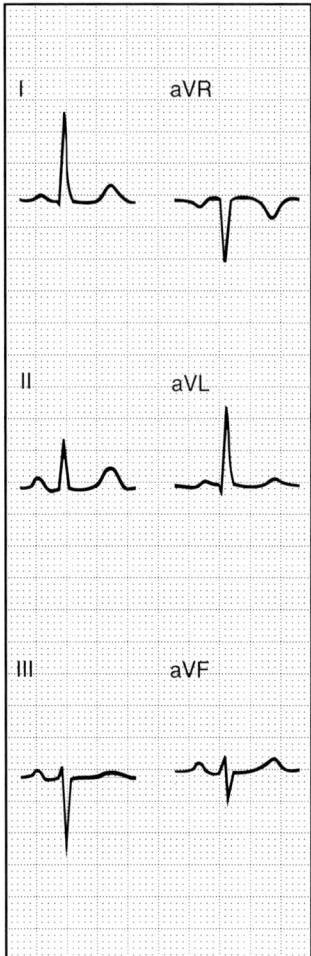

Figure 5.5. Practice tracing.

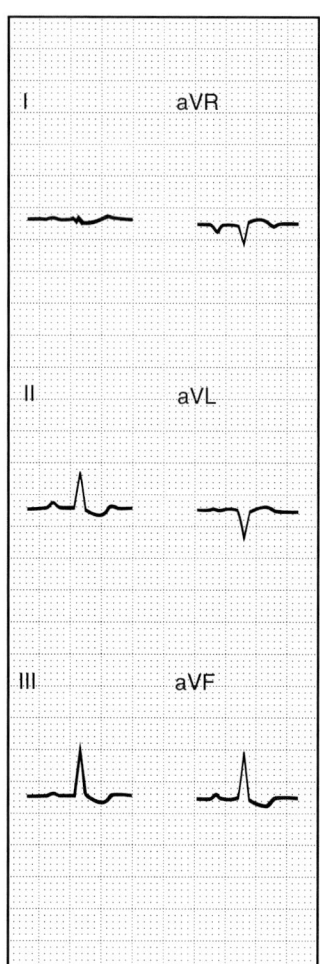

Figure 5.6. Practice tracing.

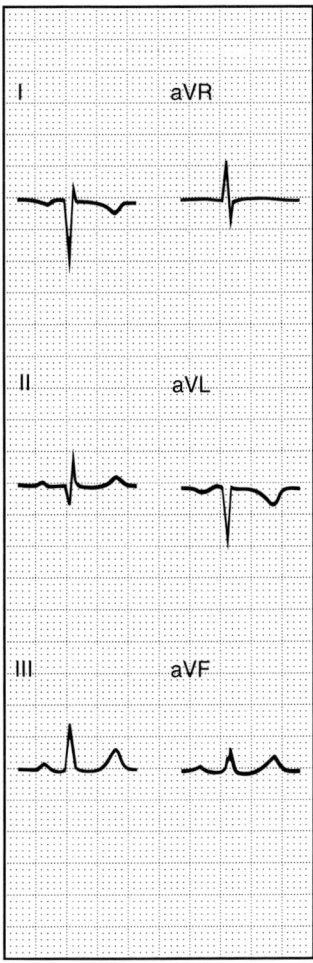

Figure 5.7. Practice tracing.

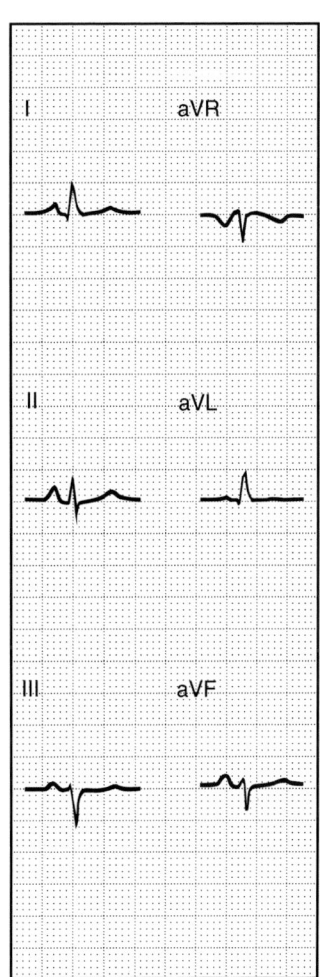

Figure 5.8. Practice tracing.

6

Intraventricular Conduction Delays: The Hemiblocks

Having just completed a study of electrical axis, we now will logically turn our attention to the so-called hemiblocks, as their diagnosis depends so heavily on marked shifts in electrical axis.

Anatomy

You will recall from Chapter 1 (Figure 1.1) that the left bundle divides very early into a left anterosuperior fascicle and a left posteroinferior fascicle. In cross-section, one can readily see that these two fascicles run toward the *anterior* and *posterior papillary muscles*, respectively (Figure 6.1). In reality, there is an additional third fascicle, called the *centriseptal fascicle*, which supplies the septum, but because it has little clinical bearing electrocardiographically, we will stick with the simpler clinical concept of two major divisions of the left bundle.

Failure of the Fascicles

As you might surmise, anything that can go wrong, will go wrong. So, of course, we can foresee that there might be occasions when, for whatever reason, one or the other (or both) of these two fascicles will fail to work properly. Failure may include delays in repolarization, so that the impulse finds the fascicle still refractory; conduction of impulses more slowly than usual; or complete inability to conduct an impulse.

When either the anterosuperior or posteroinferior fascicle fails, we say that it is "blocked," and we call the failure *hemiblock*. In everyday parlance, we shorten the names to just left anterior hemiblock (LAH) and *left posterior hemiblock (LPH)*.

Effect of Hemiblock on Sequence of Activation

Left Anterior Hemiblock

As you know from Chapter 5, any change in the sequence of activation of the ventricles will change the axis or direction of vector 3, which is our main vector of ventricular depolarization. To illustrate the impact of hemiblocks, let's begin by considering LAH.

Figure 6.1. Schematic section through the left ventricle as viewed from the patient's left (posterior axillary view) showing how the anterior and posterior fascicles of the left bundle run toward their respective papillary muscles.

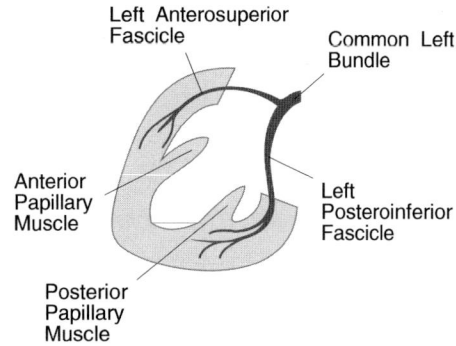

In LAH, the impulse comes down the main left bundle and the left posterior fascicle quite normally (Figure 6.2). However, the impulse finds the left anterior fascicle blocked. As a result, the posteroinferior section of the ventricle is activated first. A wave of depolarization then spreads by slow conduction from muscle fiber to muscle fiber into the portion of the ventricle that is normally served by the anterosuperior fascicle. The net result is a vector spreading superiorly through the wall of the left ventricle and shifting the axis of main ventricular depolarization counterclockwise to the left. This axis shift is so pronounced that LAH usually produces marked LAD, frequently approaching −60 degrees (Figure 6.3). Exactly how extreme the LAD is depends upon what the patient's normal axis was before developing the hemiblock.

Although vector 3 is dramatically shifted to the left, it should be readily apparent that septal depolarization is still occurring normally because the posterior fascicle is still intact, and it is the posterior fascicle that predominantly supplies the septum with Purkinje fibers. Therefore, as you will note in Figure 6.3, although lead III is now predominantly negative, there is still a small R wave present, reflecting normal septal depolarization. Note that there is still a small Q present in lead I, also, of course, reflecting normal septal depolarization.

Criteria for LAH

The diagnostic criteria, then, for isolated LAH include the following:

1. Marked LAD, frequently approaching −60 degrees
2. A small R in lead III

Figure 6.2. Left anterior hemiblock. Schematic frontal section through the anterior wall of the left ventricle, just anterior to the anterior papillary muscle. The right ventricle is not seen because it lies anterior to the left ventricle and is cut away. In this illustration, the anterior fascicle of the left bundle is blocked. As a result, depolarization is initiated by the Purkinje system of the posterior fascicle behind the posterior papillary muscle. A vector then spreads to the patient's left and superiorly into the region served by the anterosuperior fascicle, as illustrated by the arrow, producing LAD. Note that the septum will still be depolarized normally from left to right by the intact posterior fascicle.

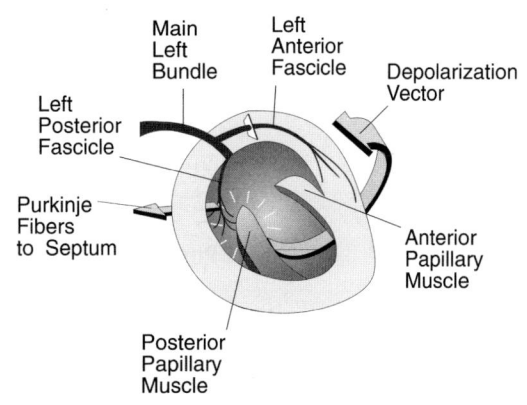

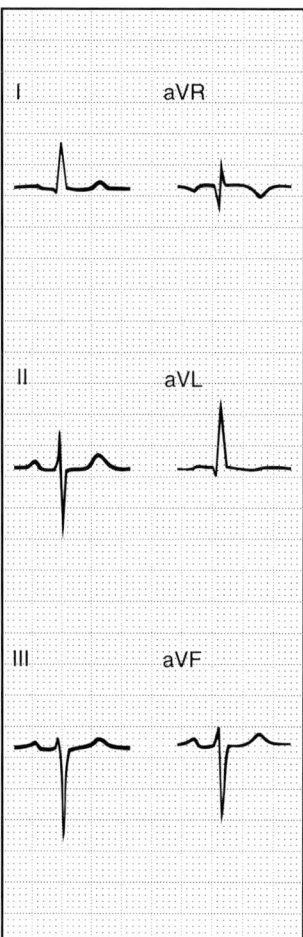

Figure 6.3. Left anterior hemiblock. Marked LAD of −60 degrees is present, as quickly confirmed by the equally biphasic QRS in lead aVR. In addition, there is a small R in lead III, and a small Q in lead I. The QRS duration is normal.

3. A small Q in lead I
4. Normal QRS duration

Why normal QRS duration? Although LAH certainly falls within the technical category of a *delay in intraventricular conduction* because it can increase QRS duration by 0.01 to 0.02 s, note in Figure 6.3 that the QRS duration is still normal. This is because, although activation of the left superior ventricle is somewhat delayed, it is a small enough area with a short enough transit time required for the wave of muscle-to-muscle depolarization that no significant prolongation of the QRS to 0.10 s or greater results.

Left Posterior Hemiblock

The story for LPH is essentially the reverse of LAH, as illustrated in Figure 6.4. The impulse travels down the anterior fascicle quite normally, but finds the posterior fascicle blocked. As a result, the anterosuperior wall of the

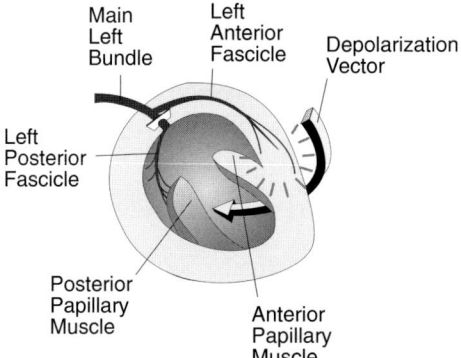

Figure 6.4. Left posterior hemiblock. Schematic frontal section through the left ventricle illustrating sequences of depolarization in LPH. The impulse descends the left anterior fascicle normally, and then spreads by slow muscle-to-muscle conduction to the right and posteriorly toward the region of the ventricle normally served by the left posterior fascicle. The net result in the frontal plane is a left-to-right vector that produces RAD. Note that in posterior hemiblock the posterior fascicle can no longer depolarize the septum. Septal depolarization therefore takes place from right to left via Purkinje fibers from the right bundle branch (not depicted).

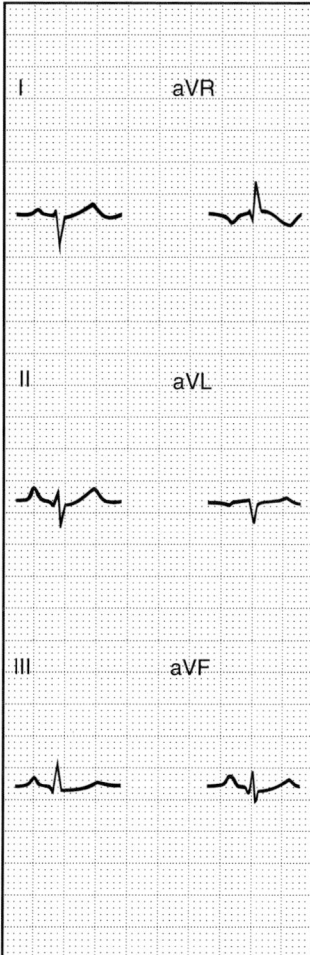

Figure 6.5. Left posterior hemiblock. Marked right axis deviation of 170 degrees is present, along with a small R in lead I, and a small Q in lead III.

left ventricle is activated first, and then a slow muscle-to-muscle wave of depolarization spreads inferiorly and to the right in the direction of the posterior papillary muscle (Figure 6.4). The net result in this instance is prominent RAD with an electrical axis that may approach +120 degrees or more, again depending on the patient's normal axis before developing hemiblock. (Figure 6.5).

But this time, because the Purkinje fibers that supply the septum are a part of the posterior fascicle and are therefore blocked, septal depolarization no longer occurs from left to right. Instead, the septum is now depolarized by the right bundle, and the result is a right-to-left vector across the septum. Thus, with LPH, we now see in Figure 6.5 a small Q in lead III, and a small R in lead I- just the opposite of what we see with LAH. As before, QRS duration remains normal.

Criteria for LPH

In summary, then, the criteria for isolated LPH are as follows:

1. RAD, often approaching +120 degrees
2. Small Q in lead III
3. Small R in lead I
4. Normal QRS duration

Confusion of LAH with Inferior Wall Myocardial Infarction

You will later learn that one of the hallmarks of AMI is the development of Q waves. In inferior wall myocardial infarction, very deep Q waves can develop in the leads that look at the inferior wall of the heart, that is, in leads II, III, and aVF (Figure 6.6).

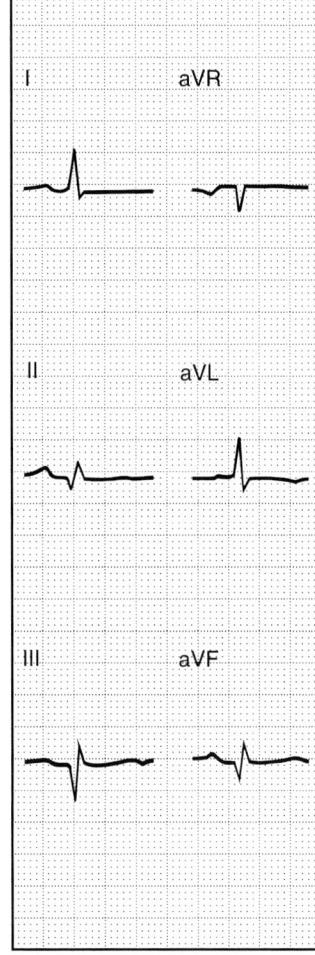

Figure 6.6. Old inferior wall myocardial infarction with Q waves in leads II, III, and aVF, and with an axis of approximately −5 degrees.

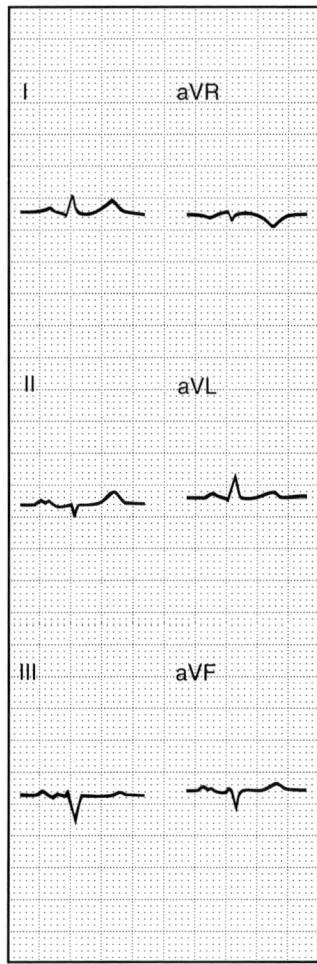

Figure 6.7. Left anterior hemiblock with deep S waves in the inferior wall (II, III, and aVF) which can be mistaken for old inferior myocardial infarction if the reader does not notice that there are actually tiny initial R waves present in leads III and aVF, and not Q waves. In addition, the LAD is more extreme, at about −50 degrees.

Because LAH produces deep S waves in leads II, III, and aVF, these S waves can sometimes be mistaken for the Q waves of inferior myocardial infarction if the reader does not notice the small R wave in front of the S wave (Figure 6.7).

In inferior wall myocardial infarction, the development of the Q wave in leads II, III, and aVF eliminates the small R in lead III that is present in LAH. Thus, the presence or absence of the small R in lead III is important in helping to distinguish an inferior wall myocardial infarction from LAH, and, for that reason, is a part of the criteria necessary to define LAH. This concept will become clearer after your study of myocardial infarction in Chapter 9.

In addition, note in Figure 6.6 that the presence of Q waves in inferior wall myocardial infarction alone does not usually produce the extreme LAD seen with LAH.

Block of Both Fascicles

We mentioned at the beginning of this chapter that it is quite possible for both the left anterior and posterior fascicles to fail to conduct an impulse. In this instance, of course, we essentially have failure of the entire left bundle, producing *LBBB*, one of the subjects of our next chapter. Combinations of RBBB and one or the other of the hemiblocks will also be discussed in Chapter 7.

Practice Tracings

Figures 6.8–6.11 on the following two pages will offer you some practice in identifying hemiblocks. The answers may be found in Chapter 14.

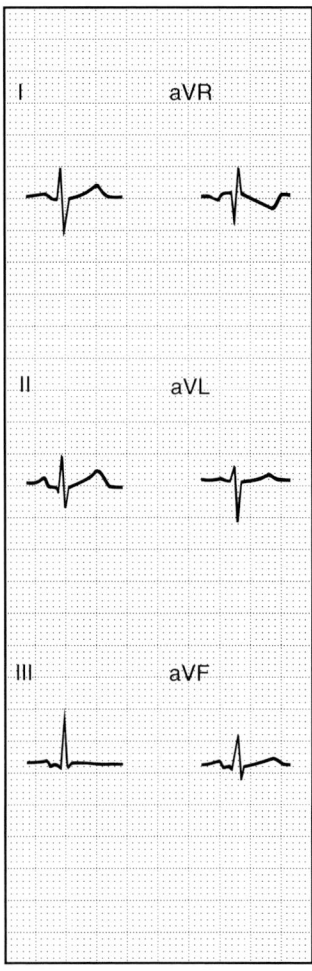

Figure 6.8. Practice tracing.

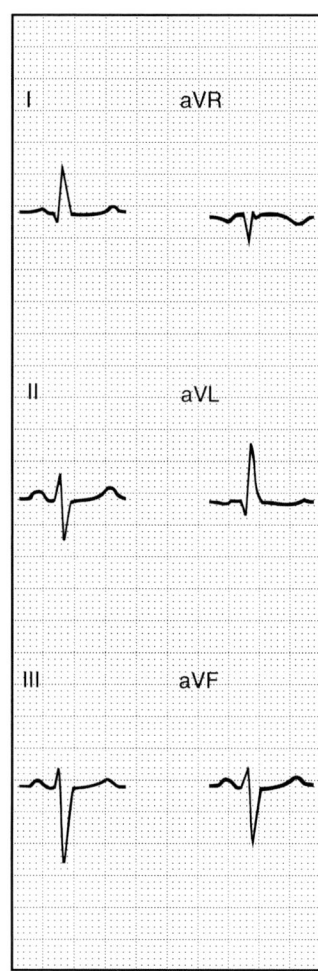

Figure 6.9. Practice tracing.

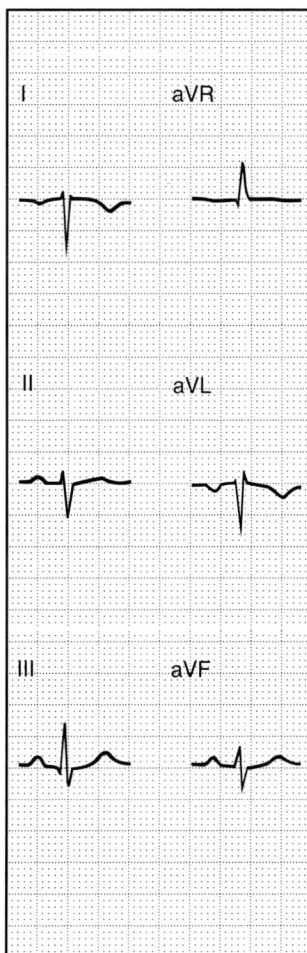

Figure 6.10. Practice tracing.

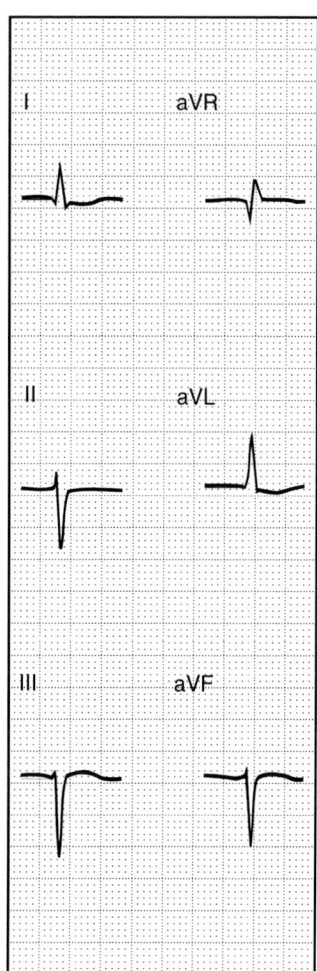

Figure 6.11. Practice tracing.

7

Intraventricular Conduction Delays: The Bundle Branch Blocks

In Chapter 6, we examined a form of delays in intraventricular conduction that did not prolong the duration of the QRS—namely the hemiblocks. In Chapter 7, we will examine more severe intraventricular conduction delays that do result in QRS prolongation—the bundle branch blocks (BBBs).

Anatomy and Pathophysiology

By now you are familiar with the specialized conduction system of the heart. *Bundle branch block* is the pattern produced when either the right bundle or the entire left bundle (both fascicles) fails to conduct an impulse normally.

As you will recall from Chapter 6, there are essentially three mechanisms for the failure of a portion of the conduction system to conduct impulses normally:

1. Delays in repolarization so that the impulse finds a portion of the conduction system still refractory
2. Reduction in the normal speed of conduction
3. Complete inability to conduct an impulse

Complete BBB

The BBBs are divided into two categories of severity, *complete* and *incomplete*. In complete BBBs, there is total failure of the affected bundle branch to conduct an impulse. The ventricle on the side of the failed bundle branch must be depolarized by the spread of a wave of depolarization through ventricular muscle from the unaffected side (Figure 7.1). Obviously, this activation of the affected ventricle by muscle-to-muscle conduction is a much slower process than rapid activation through the Purkinje fibers of a normally functioning bundle branch. In addition, there is a lot of ground to cover; essentially, an entire ventricle. The result is that, in complete BBBs, the QRS duration is prolonged to at least 0.12 seconds or greater.

Figure 7.1. Right bundle branch block. The ventricle on the side of the failed bundle must be depolarized by the spread of a wave of depolarization from the nonaffected side (arrow).

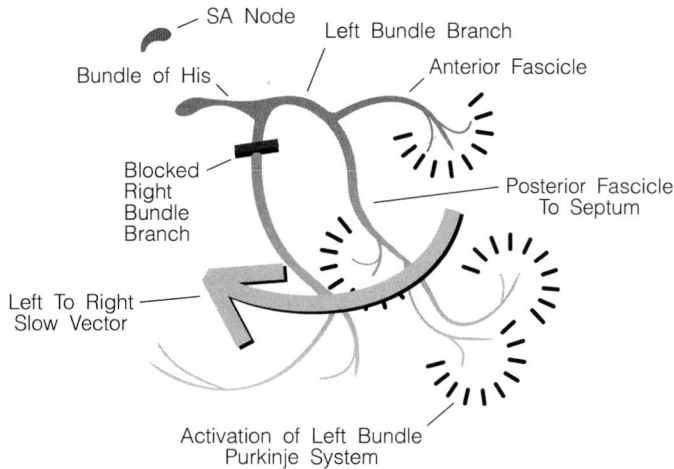

Incomplete BBB

Sometimes, the blocked bundle branch is not really totally blocked, but merely conducts the impulse more slowly than usual. This delays depolarization of the affected ventricle long enough for a wave of depolarization to begin spreading over muscle across from the unaffected side. In the meantime, the impulse also finally travels down the partially blocked bundle branch and reaches the Purkinje fibers on the affected side. The result is that part of the muscle on the affected side is activated by the conduction system and part is activated by the slow wave of depolarization spreading over muscle from the normal, or unaffected, side (Figure 7.2). This produces a QRS that is not quite as wide as in complete BBB, but is wider than normal. In other words, QRS duration in incomplete BBB is between 0.10 and 0.12 s.

Figure 7.2. Incomplete RBBB. The impulse comes down the left bundle normally, initiating normal depolarization of the left ventricle (Event 1). Next, a slow vector of muscle-to-muscle depolarization begins to spread into the right ventricle (Event 2). Finally, the delayed impulse coming down the right bundle reaches the Purkinje fibers (Event 3). The net result is that the right ventricle is depolarized by both the slow vector spreading from the left ventricle and the delayed impulse coming down the right bundle. This produces a QRS that is intermediate in duration; i.e., between 0.10 and 0.12 s.

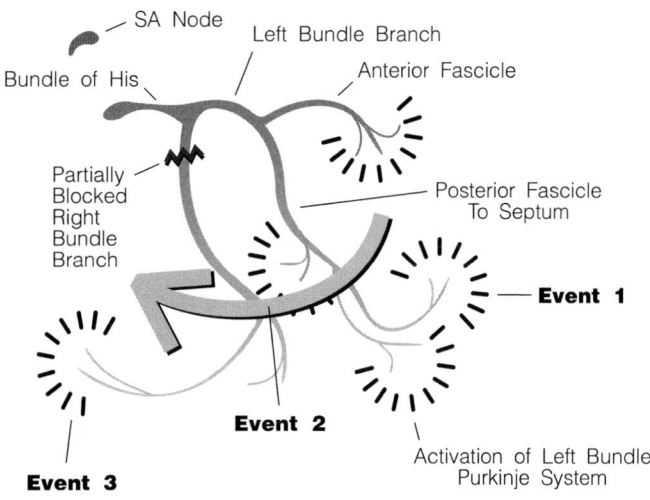

Looking for BBBs in the V Leads

Although the QRS is prolonged in all leads in BBB, you will see very shortly that particularly characteristic patterns are produced in the precordial leads that make it very easy to distinguish RBBB from LBBB. For this reason, most of our discussion will concern the impact of BBB on the V leads.

Of course, there is also reason to examine the limb leads in BBB, primarily to determine electrical axis. You will learn that either RAD or LAD can be seen with both RBBB and LBBB, and that these axis shifts do have some significance.

Complete RBBB

Now let's look at some specifics. You will note in Figure 7.3 that RBBB reverses our normal pattern of a predominantly negative QRS in lead V_1. Instead, we see an upright QRS with an RSR′. Now let's see if we can figure out what produces this pattern. In RBBB, the impulse goes down the left bundle quite normally and activates the septum and then the left ventricle. Because the septum is depolarized normally, we can expect our initial QRS deflection to be quite normal and to produce an initial R wave in lead V_1 and a normal initial Q wave in leads V_5 and V_6.

Next, we see the beginning of an S wave in lead V_1 and an R wave in lead V_6. This reflects normal depolarization of the left ventricle. However, at this point (which is actually quite late in the QRS), our wave of depolarization in the left ventricle begins to slowly travel across muscle into the right ventricle and, therefore, toward lead V_1. This produces a second positive deflection in lead V_1 (the R′) and a late S wave in leads V_5 and V_6. Note that the slowness of this process is reflected by the fact that the R′ in lead V_1 and the S wave in leads V_5 and V_6 are quite wide and account for the increase in our QRS duration to 0.12 s or greater.

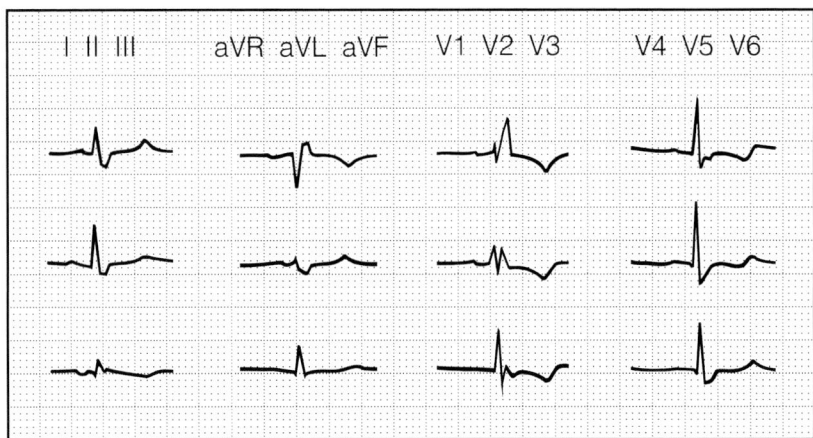

Figure 7.3. Right bundle branch block showing the characteristic RSR′ pattern in the right precordial leads (V_1 and V_2), and a prominent wide S wave in the lateral precordial leads (V_5 and V_6).

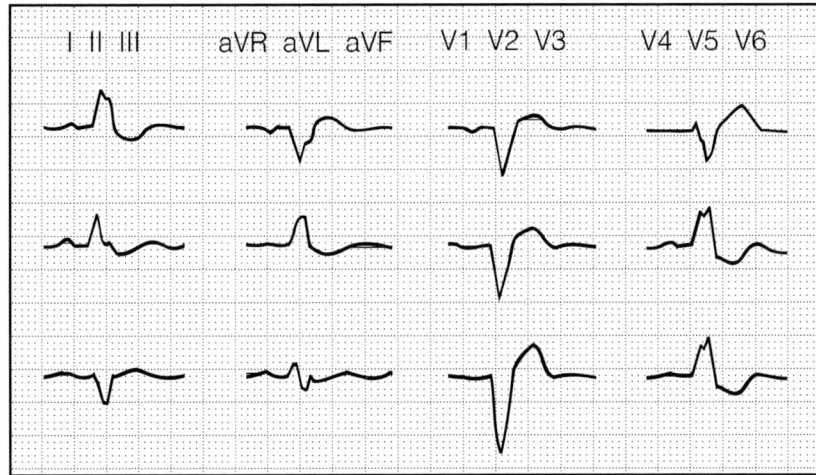

Figure 7.4. LBBB showing a deep QS in the right precordial leads (V$_1$ and V$_2$) and the typical RSR' in the left precordial leads.

We can summarize the pattern of RBBB, then, by saying that it produces an RSR' (an upright M-shaped pattern) on the right side in lead V$_1$ and a prominent, wide S on the left side in leads V$_5$ and V$_6$. You will see that LBBB produces a very similar pattern, but in reverse.

Complete LBBB

In Figure 7.4, you will see the pattern of LBBB, and will note that, indeed, it is the reverse (although not a mirror image) of RBBB, in the sense that it produces an upright "M" shaped pattern (this time on the left) in leads V$_5$ and V$_6$, and a deep, negative QS on the right in leads V$_1$ and V$_2$.

In LBBB, the impulse, of course, finds the left bundle blocked and goes down the right bundle (Figure 7.5). The septum, as usual, is the first part of

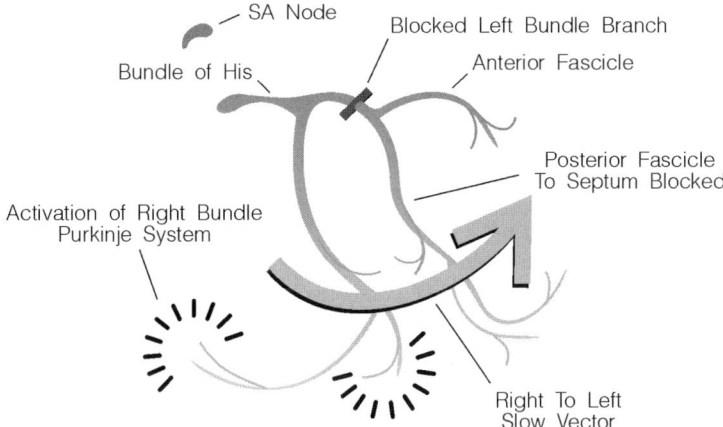

Figure 7.5. Left bundle branch block. The left ventricle is depolarized by a large slow vector that is initiated by the intact right bundle and spreads from right to left, into the left ventricle.

the ventricles to be activated, but because the left bundle is blocked, the septum is now activated by Purkinje fibers from the right bundle, producing a right-to-left vector across the septum. Thus, the first deflection of our QRS will be negative in lead V_1 and positive in lead V_6. Our normal initial R in lead V_1 becomes a Q, and our normal initial Q in lead V_6 becomes an R.

Next, the right ventricle is activated, but usually does not produce an R wave in V_1, possibly for two reasons. The first is that the vector of right ventricular depolarization traveling from endocardium to epicardium toward lead V_1 is partially counterbalanced by the continuing right-to-left vector in the opposite direction through the septum with its greater muscle mass.

The second explanation is that upon normal activation of the right ventricle, a large slow vector immediately begins to spread into the larger mass of the left ventricle across muscle from right to left, also helping to counterbalance what would usually be our normal small R wave in lead V_1.

Nevertheless, it is worthwhile to note that, occasionally, the right ventricular forces spreading from endocardium to epicardium are still strong enough in LBBB to produce a tiny R wave in leads V_1 and V_2 (Figure 7.6).

Finally, the right ventricle finishes depolarizing before the slow wave of depolarization has finished spreading from right to left across the left ventricle. This leaves the vector spreading through the left ventricle unopposed and completes the wide, deep QS that we see in lead V_1 in LBBB.

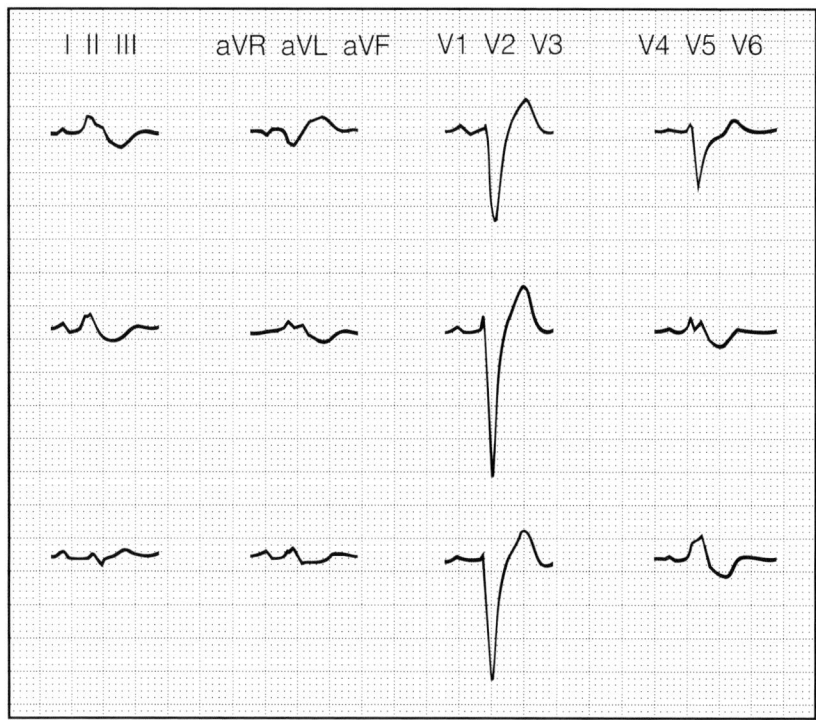

Figure 7.6. Left bundle branch block with small R waves in V_1 and V_2.

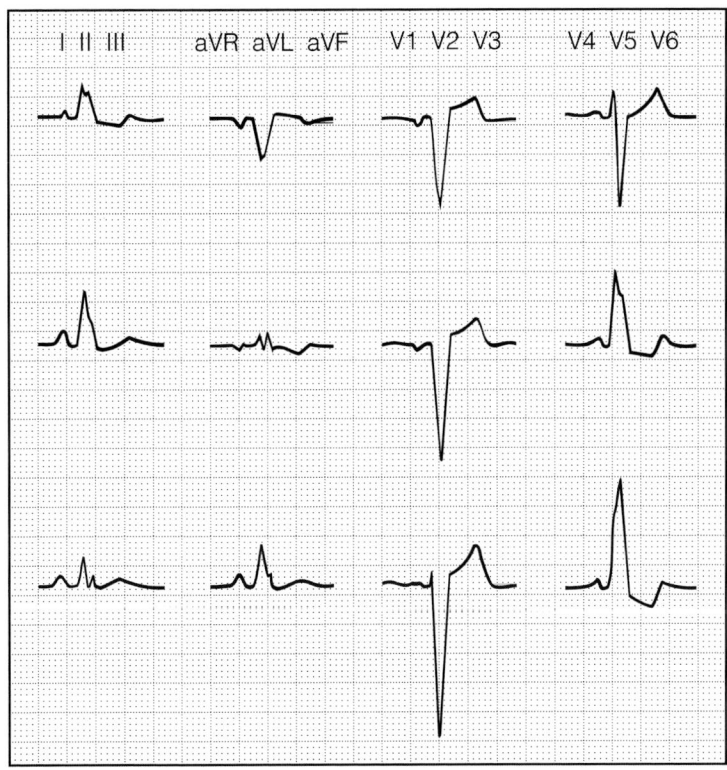

Figure 7.7. Left bundle branch block showing a monophasic QRS in V_5 and V_6, without the characteristic RSR′ pattern.

While producing a deep QS in lead V_1, these same right-to-left forces are producing a wide positive deflection in leads V_5 and V_6. Usually, the QRS in the left precordial leads (V_5 and V_6) is *monophasic*, as seen in Figure 7.7, meaning that it goes in only one direction (in this case upwardly without a negative deflection). However, sometimes the right ventricular forces will be strong enough to produce a small S in the middle of the QRS followed by an R′, thus, again producing an M-shaped pattern on the left as in Figure 7.4.

BBBs, ST Segments, and T Waves

You will note that in all of the examples of BBB that you have seen so far, the ST segments and T waves appear abnormal. Along with the abnormalities of depolarization in BBB come abnormalities of repolarization. Thus, it is characteristic of BBB that the T waves are usually inscribed in the opposite direction from the terminal portion of the QRS. This is because, as you learned earlier, it is the terminal portion of the QRS that reflects the large, slow, abnormal vector of muscle-to-muscle depolarization that is characteristic of BBB.

Note that also the ST segments are typically slurred into the inverted T waves. These ST and T wave changes are called *secondary changes* because they occur as the result of the intraventricular conduction delay rather than as a primary reflection of some other myocardial abnormality.

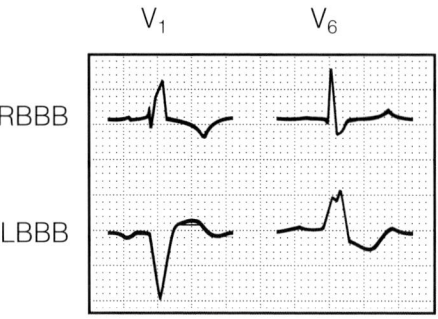

Figure 7.8. Comparison chart of RBBB and LBBB as seen in leads V_1 and V_6.

Summary of Findings in BBB

Figure 7.8 compares typical RBBB with LBBB. Note that RBBB displays the upright "M" on the right side of the precordial leads (V_1), and LBBB displays the upright "M" on the left side. Thus, if you simply remember *right on the right* and *left on the left*, you can easily distinguish between the two. Note also that the two are very easy to distinguish in lead V_1 alone. Right BBB in V_1 is upright and M-shaped, and LBBB in lead V_1 is quite the opposite, with a deep QS.

Incomplete BBB and Nonspecific Intraventricular Conduction Delays

Figure 7.9 shows a tracing with an RSR′ in V_2 that is typical of RBBB, but with a narrower QRS duration of 0.10 s or greater and <0.12 s You will also note that in this tracing the QRSs are less bizarre, and there are fewer

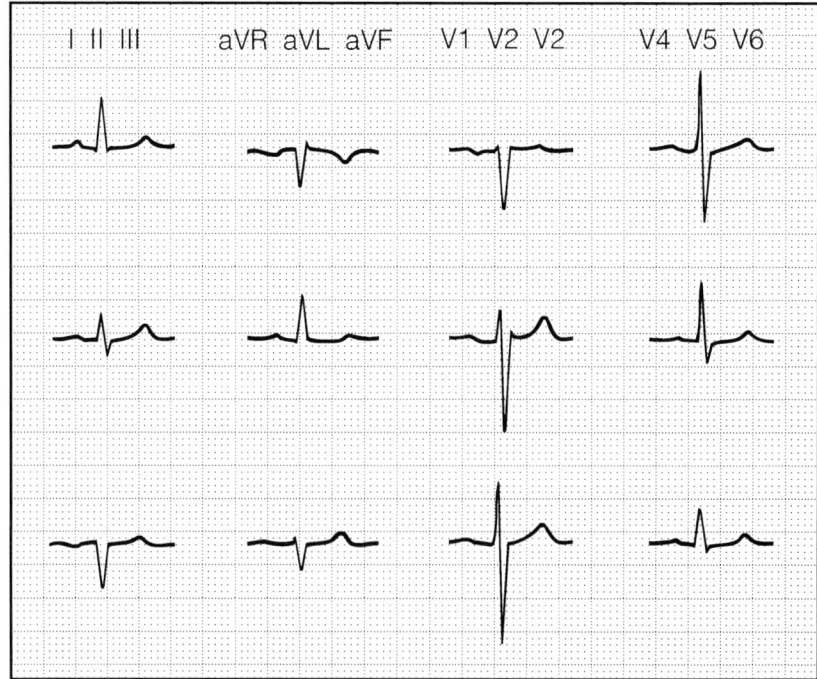

Figure 7.9. Incomplete RBBB displaying an RSR′ in lead V_2, and mild QRS prolongation with a QRS duration of 0.104 s, but less than the 0.12 s required for complete BBB. Note that few secondary ST and T wave changes are present.

Figure 7.10. Incomplete LBBB showing a QRS duration of 0.116 s with either no R wave or tiny R waves in the right precordial leads (poor R wave progression) and a deep S. The QRS is upright on the left, with only mild secondary ST and T wave changes.

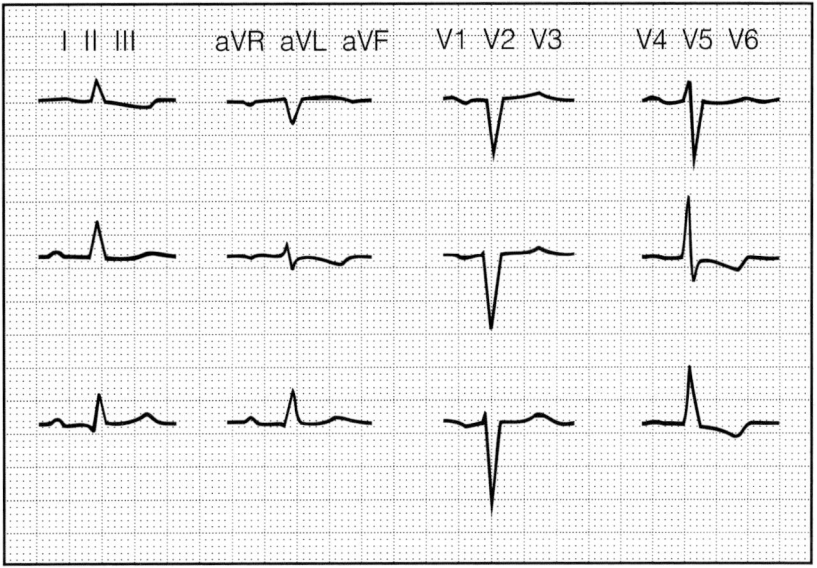

secondary ST and T wave changes. This tracing falls into the category of incomplete RBBB, which was referred to earlier.

The usual pattern of complete LBBB is altered in similar ways in incomplete LBBB (Figure 7.10). These findings reflect delay in conduction of the impulse by the affected bundle branch, rather than total failure.

Not infrequently, one sees a tracing with QRS prolongation of 0.10 s or greater that does not have a pattern typical of either RBBB or LBBB. Electrocardiographers frequently refer to such tracings as showing an *intraventricular conduction delay*, which is *nonspecific* (Figure 7.11).

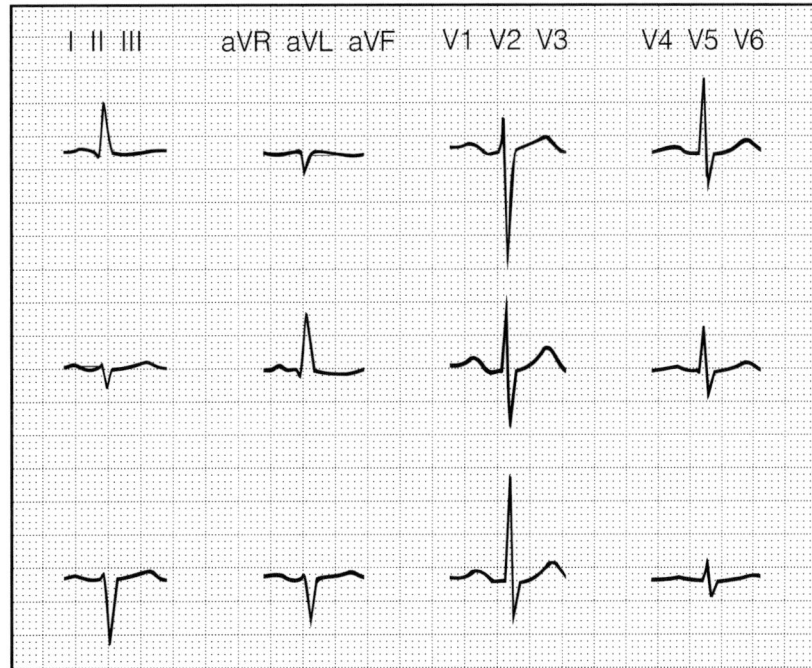

Figure 7.11. Nonspecific intraventricular conduction delay with QRS duration of 0.108 s. Pattern in the V leads is not typical of either incomplete RBBB or LBBB.

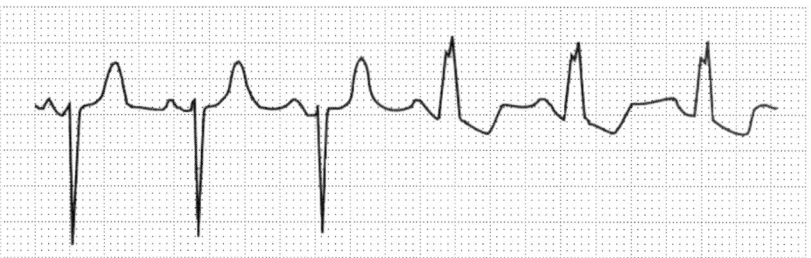

Figure 7.12. Rate-dependent BBB. This patient switches conduction to a RBBB pattern when his rate reaches approximately 85. This rhythm strip is recorded in lead V$_1$.

Intermittent BBB and Supraventricular Aberrancy

If one of the bundle branches repolarizes slightly slower than the other, it would be possible to find a heart rate that would be slow enough to allow one bundle branch adequate time for repolarization, but too fast to allow the other bundle branch adequate time for repolarization. Such a circumstance produces what is called a *rate dependent BBB*. As soon as the R-to-R intervals become shorter than the time required for the repolarization of the slower of the two bundle branches, the patient's tracing switches from normal conduction to a BBB pattern, as seen in Figure 7.12.

Conversely, when the patient's heart rate slows enough to allow both bundle branches adequate time for repolarization, the tracing will switch back to a pattern of normal conduction with a narrow QRS. For example, if the right bundle branch requires 600 ms to repolarize, as soon as the R-to-R interval becomes <600 ms, a RBBB pattern will appear. When the R-to-R interval becomes >600 ms, the RBBB pattern will disappear. This example is actually quite practical because, in most of us, it is the right bundle branch that is the slowest to repolarize. Thus, most patients who display a rate-dependent BBB develop a RBBB pattern when their rate becomes too fast.

It is exactly the same phenomenon that produces aberrant conduction of premature supraventricular beats. If, for instance, the impulse of a premature atrial contraction reaches the bundle branches in the aforementioned patient example in less than the 600 ms required for repolarization, it will find the right bundle still refractory, and the premature atrial contraction will be aberrantly conducted with a RBBB pattern (Figure 7.13).

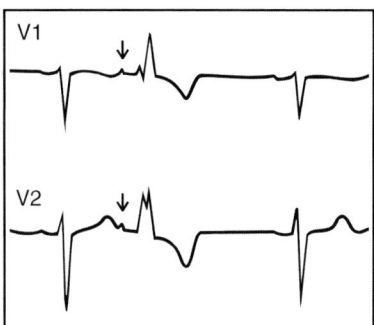

Figure 7.13. An aberrantly conducted PAC, as seen in leads V$_1$ and V$_2$, which finds the right bundle branch still refractory and, thus, produces a RBBB pattern. The PAC is marked with an arrow.

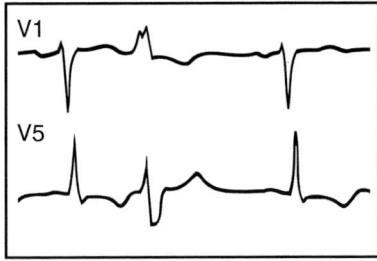

Figure 7.14. Premature ventricular contraction arising from the left ventricle, producing a RBBB pattern.

Thus, when it is difficult to determine whether an aberrantly conducted beat is a supraventricular beat with aberrancy, or a PVC, the presence of a RBBB pattern makes it slightly more likely to be supraventricular because, in most of us, the right bundle repolarizes slightly more slowly than the left.

Relationship of BBB Patterns to PVCs and Paced Beats

Now that you understand why the QRS is prolonged to 0.12s or greater in BBB, you can also understand why PVCs are always 0.12s or greater. It is, again, because the ventricles are being activated by the slow process of muscle-to-muscle conduction, rather than being rapidly depolarized through the Purkinje system.

You can also now understand that we can frequently determine the general location from which a PVC is arising by looking at its pattern in the precordial leads. A PVC arising in the left ventricle will produce a vector slowly spreading to the right ventricle, and will, thus, produce a pattern similar to the pattern of RBBB (Figure 7.14).

On the other hand, a wave of depolarization arising from a PVC in the right ventricle will slowly spread toward the left ventricle, simulating the pattern of LBBB (Figure 7.15).

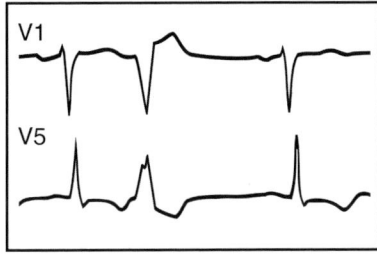

Figure 7.15. Premature ventricular contraction arising from the right ventricle, producing a LBBB pattern.

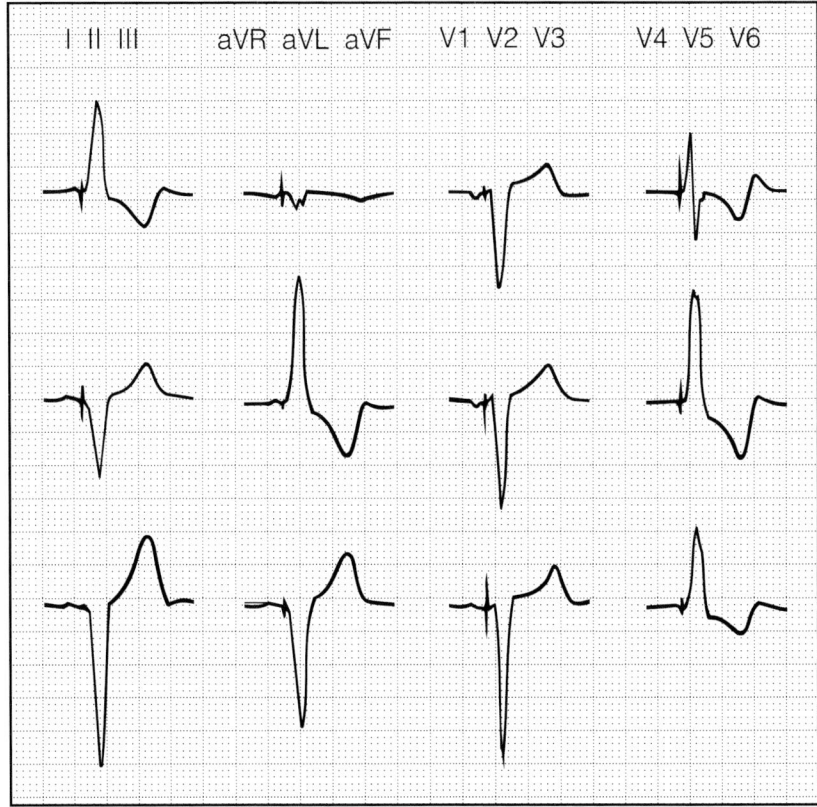

Figure 7.16. Paced beats from a pacemaker that is placed, as usual, in the apex of the right ventricle, producing a LBBB pattern.

Exactly the same phenomenon occurs when a pacemaker fires from the apex of the right ventricle. Electrocardiographically, it produces a similar pattern to a PVC arising from the right ventricle. Pacemakers that are properly placed in the right ventricle therefore produce a LBBB pattern (Figure 7.16).

Bifascicular and Trifascicular Block

Now that you have completed study of both the hemiblocks and the BBBs, it may have occurred to you that there would be situations in which there could be combinations of BBB and hemiblock. Indeed, this is the case.

If we consider that there are normally three major final or distal routes for conduction of an impulse to the ventricles (the right bundle branch plus the two left bundle fascicles), we can easily envision that there could be block present in two of the three, or in all three pathways (fascicles).

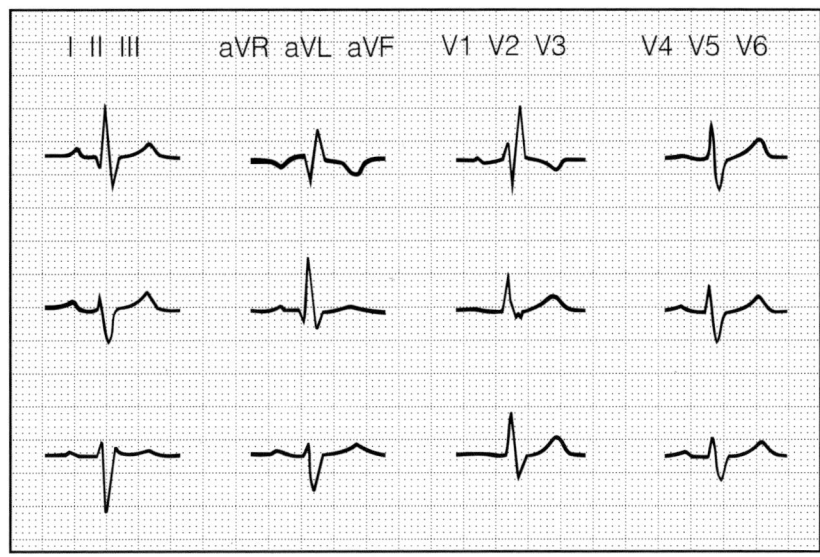

Figure 7.17. Right bundle branch block and LAH. Tracing displays RBBB with extreme left axis deviation (−55 degrees), a small Q in lead I, and a small R in lead III.

Figure 7.17 shows a tracing with not only RBBB but also with extreme LAD, a small Q in lead I, and a small R in lead III. This patient has both RBBB and LAH.

Figure 7.18 again shows a tracing with typical RBBB in the precordial leads, but, in this case, with extreme RAD, with a small R in lead I and a small

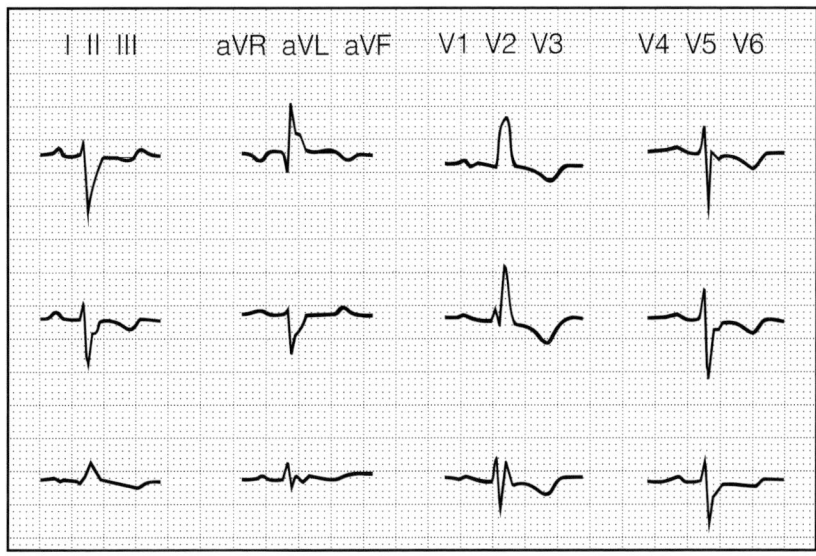

Figure 7.18. Right bundle branch block and LPH. Tracing displays RBBB with extreme right axis deviation (−175 degrees), a small R in lead I, and a very small Q in lead III.

Q in lead III. This represents the combination of RBBB and LPH. In actuality, this is the most common presentation of LPH. Isolated LPH without accompanying RBBB is very rare.

Thus, both tracings display a block of two of the three pathways, or fascicles, for impulse conduction to the ventricles, and both fall into the category of what some people call *bifascicular block*. Notice, however, that both tracings have a normal PR interval, which indicates that the impulse is getting down the remaining functioning fascicle on time. Left BBB alone is also considered to be an example of bifascicular block because both the anterior and posterior left fascicles are blocked.

As you have undoubtedly surmised by now, the term *trifascicular block* indicates either partial or complete block in all three major fascicles. Obviously, if all three fascicles are completely blocked, no impulse will reach the ventricles and, in such instances, complete AV block (third-degree block) will be present.

On the other hand, if two of the three fascicles are completely blocked, but the remaining fascicle is only partially blocked, or if there is a delay in the AV node, then we could expect to see any of our examples of bifascicular block and, in addition, a prolonged PR interval (first-degree block). Thus, if Figure 7.17 showed a PR interval of 0.20 s or greater, in addition to RBBB and LAH, we would have an example of trifascicular block. Complete LBBB with a prolonged PR interval would also be an example of trifascicular block because there would be delay in the impulse coming down the remaining functioning right bundle branch.

In summary, then, trifascicular block is present whenever we see a bifascicular block in addition to first-degree or higher AV block, which is summarized as follows:

Bifascicular Block

1. RBBB with LAH
2. RBBB with LPH
3. LBBB

Trifascicular Block

1. RBBB, LAH, and first-degree or higher AV block
2. RBBB, LPH, and first-degree or higher AV block
3. LBBB, and first-degree or higher AV block
4. Complete (third-degree) AV block

Practice Tracings

Figures 7.19–7.22 will offer you some practice in interpreting the BBBs. The answers may be found in Chapter 14.

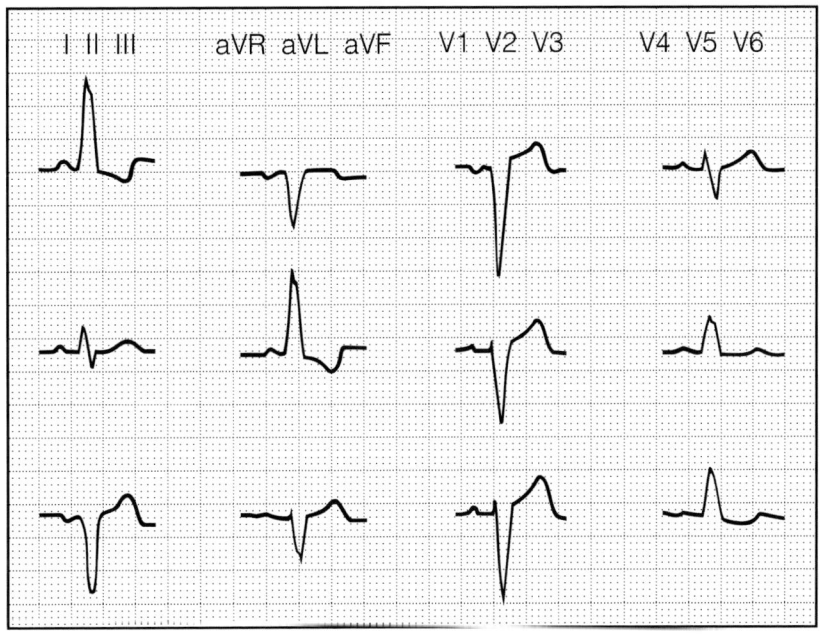

Figure 7.19. Practice tracing.

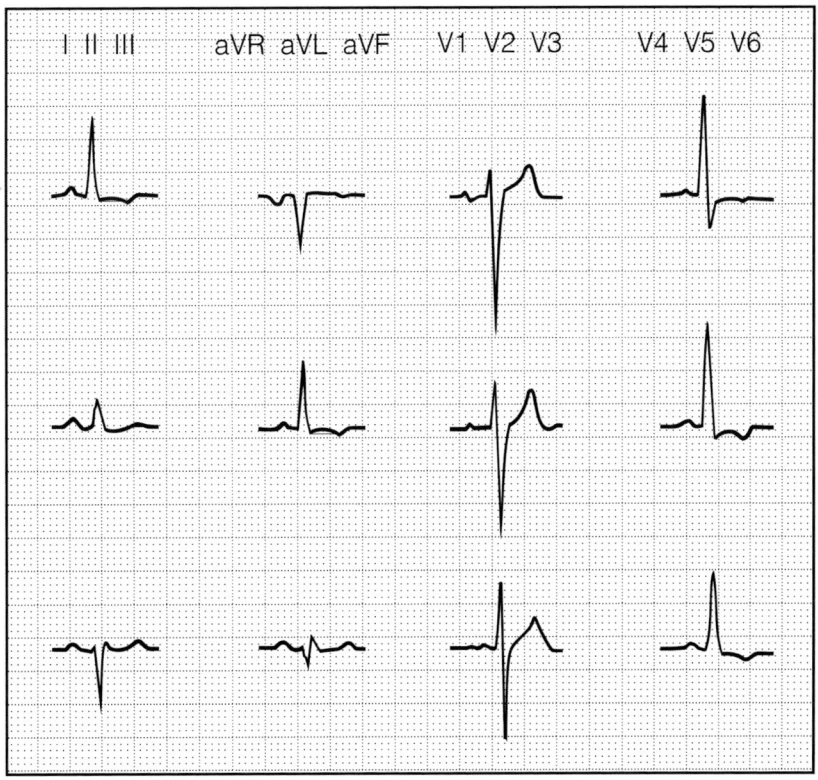

Figure 7.20. Practice tracing.

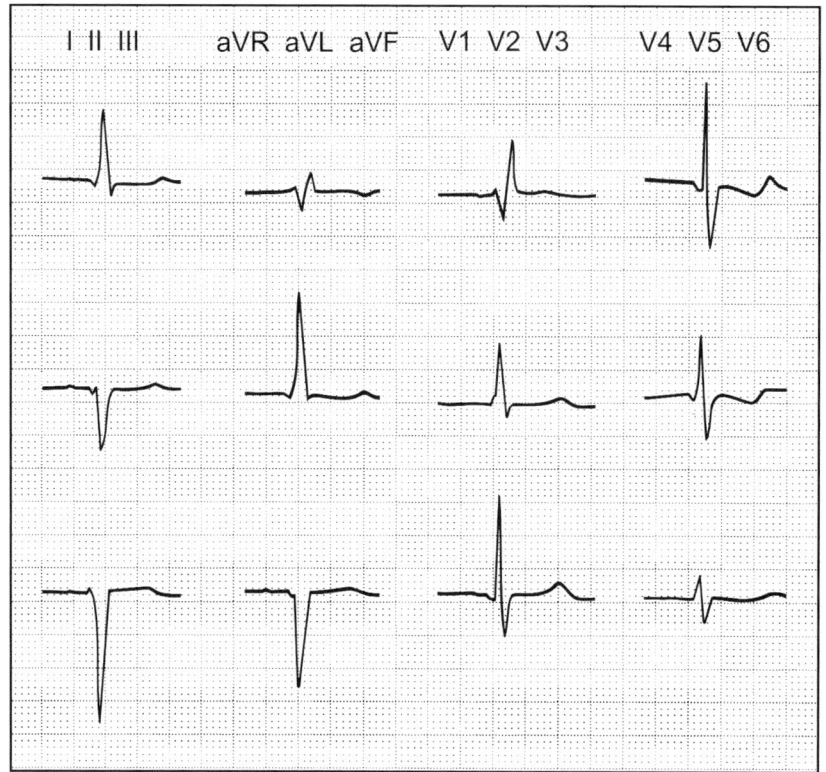

Figure 7.21. Practice tracing.

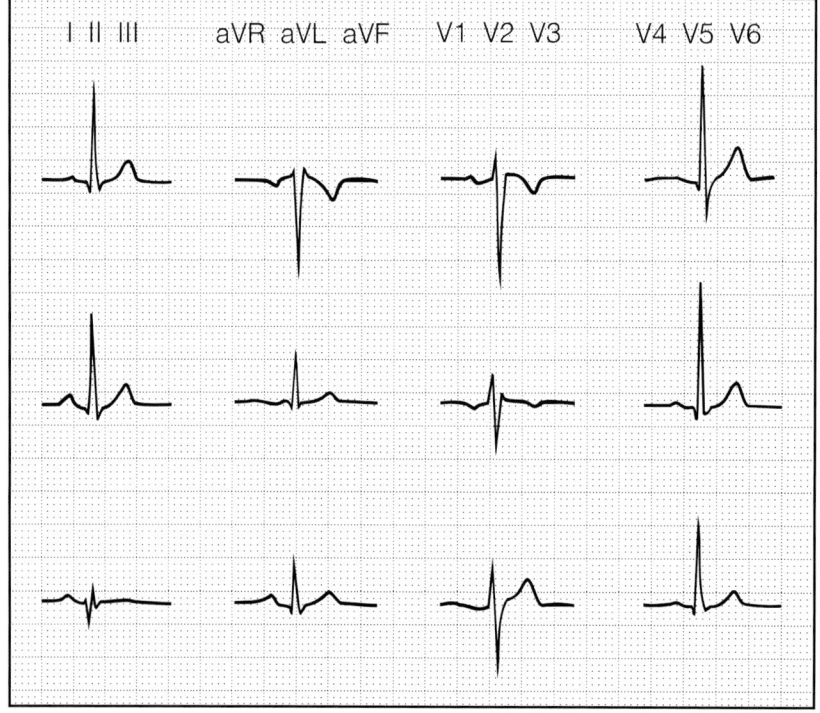

Figure 7.22. Practice tracing.

Chamber Enlargement

In this chapter, we will examine the changes elicited in the ECG by muscular hypertrophy of the ventricles.

Pathophysiology

Like any muscle, when called upon to work harder than is normally required, cardiac muscle will enlarge, or *hypertrophy*. The cause is typically either an increased resistance to outflow of blood from the chamber (as in stenosis of a valve or hypertension), or the requirement to handle increased volumes of blood (as in regurgitation of blood across an incompletely closed valve or in many forms of congenital heart disease).

The nature of the increased work is frequently that of generating higher pressures within the chamber during systole. In addition, diastolic pressures are also frequently elevated because of either a diminished *ejection fraction* (the percentage of blood ejected from the chamber with each squeeze) or increased diastolic volumes of blood (as in regurgitation). The net result is an increased muscle mass of the affected chamber.

Force Vectors in Chamber Enlargement

Many of the ECG changes caused by hypertrophy of cardiac muscle can be deduced from your knowledge of the behavior of cardiac force vectors. You already know, for example, that the larger the muscle mass, the larger the force vector and, therefore, the greater the voltage in the ECG. We could surmise that the QRS would show excessive voltage in ventricular hypertrophy.

In addition, you know that changes in the wall thickness of either the right or left ventricle could change the direction of the vector of main ventricular depolarization. We could also surmise, then, that we could see a change in electrical axis with ventricular hypertrophy.

Finally, it is logical that the greater the muscle mass, the longer it takes for a wave of depolarization to traverse that muscle mass. So we could again surmise that it would be possible to see slightly increased QRS duration in the presence of ventricular hypertrophy. Of course, all of these features may be seen in ventricular hypertrophy.

Left Ventricular Hypertrophy

In LVH, the muscle mass of the left ventricle enlarges. This tilts the main vector of ventricular depolarization more toward the left ventricle and, of course, increases its magnitude. As a result, the S wave in V_1 becomes deeper, and the R wave in the lateral precordial leads (V_5 and V_6) becomes taller. It also follows that the electrical axis may be shifted more toward the left, often, but not always, resulting in LAD. Increased amplitude of the R wave is also frequently seen in limb leads I or aVL.

Figure 8.1 shows the ECG of a 38-year-old white male with longstanding severe hypertension. Note that the S wave in lead V_1 is 31-mm-deep, and the R wave in lead V_4 is 30-mm-tall.

Many different voltage criteria for LVH have been proposed, but most electrocardiographers would agree that LVH is likely if the S wave in V_1 or V_2 or

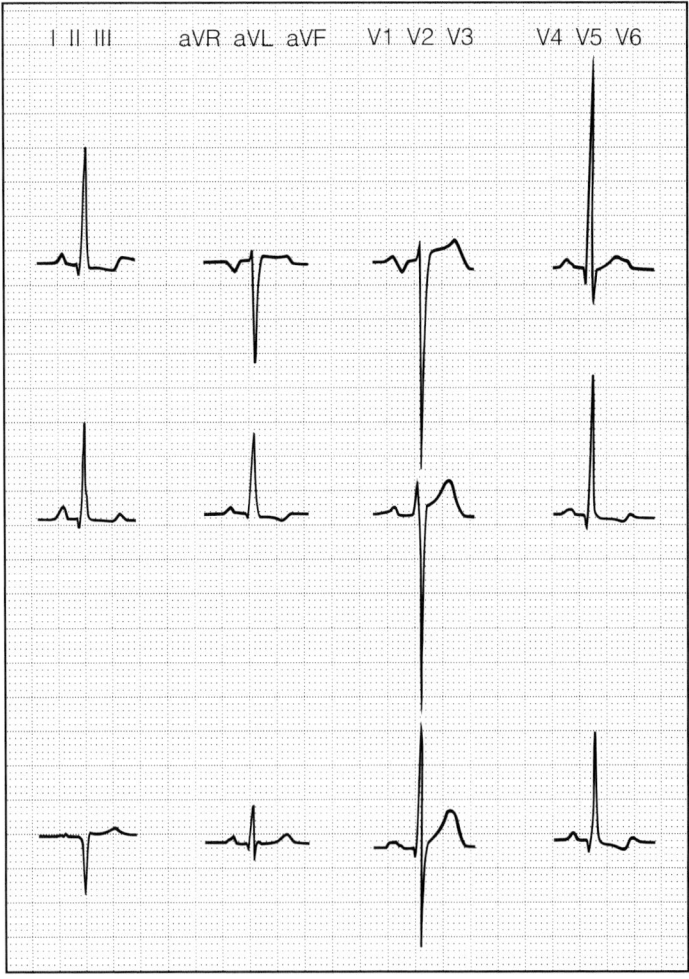

Figure 8.1. Electrocardiograph of a 38-year-old male with long-standing severe hypertension and LVH. Note the deep S wave in V_1 and V_2, and the tall R wave in V_4 exceeding 30 mm, a QRS duration at the upper limits of normal at 0.09 s, and borderline left axis deviation at 0 degrees.

the R wave in V_5 or V_6, reaches 30 mm or more in magnitude. As always, there are many normal variants among humans. Individuals with thin chest walls (children in particular) and individuals who are the size of professional basketball players may have >30 mm of QRS voltage in the absence of LVH.

QRS duration in LVH is usually only mildly increased, if at all, toward the upper limits of normal, between 0.09 and 0.10 s. This is because, although the wall of the ventricle is thicker, the wall is still being depolarized by impulses spreading through the rather rapidly conducting Purkinje system. The function of the Purkinje system is the greater determining factor in QRS duration. Figure 8.1 shows a QRS duration of 0.09 s.

Certain changes in the ST and T waves can also develop in LVH, usually most prominently in the lateral precordial leads (V_5 and V_6), but also in those limb leads toward which the main vector of depolarization is traveling (electrical axis). As hypertrophy progresses, downsloping ST depression and T wave inversion can occur, which, in the fully developed pattern, is called *left ventricular strain*. Figure 8.2 shows a fully developed strain pattern in which the ST depression is typically *upwardly convex*, with a gentle transition into an inverted T wave. These ST and T wave changes are called *secondary* because they are secondary to the LVH, rather than directly reflecting

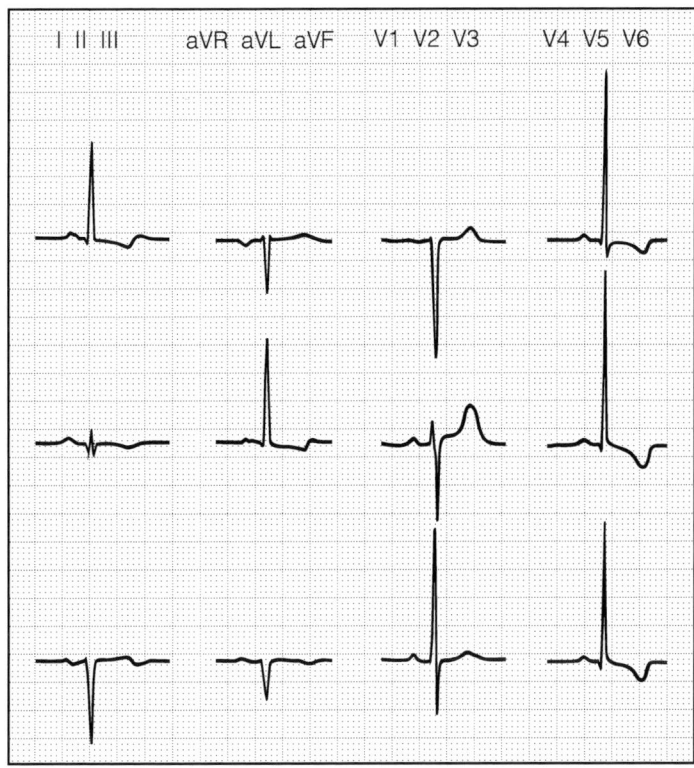

Figure 8.2. Fully developed LVH with a strain pattern. Note that the ST depression is upwardly convex and gently transitions to an inverted T. This patient also meets voltage criteria of 30 mm in V_5, and LAD with an axis of −27 degrees.

another primary myocardial abnormality. As you will learn later, the strain pattern can be confused with ST and T wave changes caused by myocardial ischemia, myocardial infarction, and other miscellaneous conditions, such as digitalis effect.

Summary of Criteria for LVH

None of the aforementioned criteria, taken alone, is a reliable indicator for LVH. You will often see electrocardiographic interpretations that read something like "LVH by voltage criteria alone." This is the electrocardiographer's way of saying that although voltage criteria are present for LVH, there are no other criteria present, and he cannot guarantee that LVH really exists in this patient.

Conversely, LVH may be present without all of the electrocardiographic criteria being met. In other words, the criteria have both *low specificity and low sensitivity* for LVH. The more criteria that are present, therefore, the more likely it is that LVH is present. The following is a summary of things to look for in trying to diagnose LVH by ECG:

1. S wave V_1 or V_2 or R wave V_5 or V_6 of 30 mm or greater.
2. LAD
3. QRS duration upper limit of normal
4. Shift in the ST segment or T wave (strain pattern) V_5 and V_6

Right Ventricular Hypertrophy

We turn our attention now to the right ventricle, where all of the same principles apply. A major difference, however, is that the right ventricle has a much smaller muscle mass to begin with than the left ventricle. Therefore, in order for the right ventricle to surpass the left ventricle in size and shift our vectors substantially to the right, it has to hypertrophy rather massively. This means that, again, our ECG criteria are not going to be very sensitive indicators of early RVH. This also accounts for the fact that full-blown RVH on an electrocardiogram is relatively rare, especially in adults.

In RVH, as the right ventricular muscle mass increases, the direction of our main vector of ventricular depolarization naturally shifts progressively toward the right. This produces a taller than normal R wave in the right-side precordial leads (V_1 and V_2). As you would guess, this also produces a fairly deep S wave in the left-side precordial leads (V_5 and V_6) (Figure 8.3).

In fact, the R wave in lead V_1 actually becomes taller than the S wave is deep. If we divide the amplitude of the R wave in lead V_1 by the amplitude of the S wave in V_1, we normally get a number of <1.0. This is called the *R-to-S ratio* (Figure 8.4). In RVH, however, the R-to-S ratio becomes >1.0 because of the exceptionally tall R wave. In other words, the usual pattern of

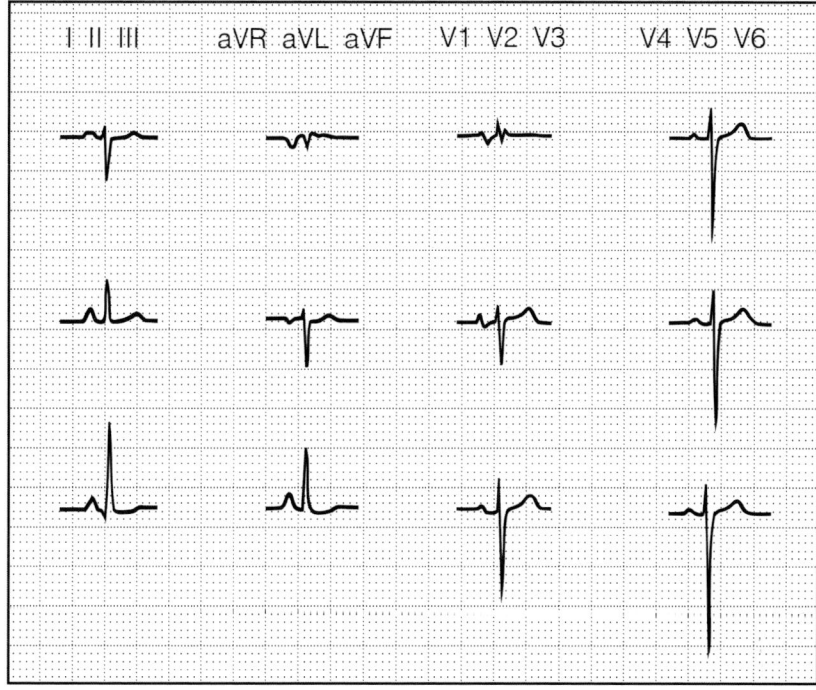

Figure 8.3. Right ventricular hypertrophy, with a tall R wave in the right-sided precordial leads and a deep S in the left-sided precordial leads.

the R wave becoming progressively taller across the precordium from right to left is reversed.

You will recall that in RBBB, we see a similar pattern of a tall R wave in V_1 and a deep S wave in V_6 (see Figure 7.3). To avoid confusing RVH with RBBB, we must therefore insist that the QRS be of normal duration when diagnosing RVH. The QRS duration can be in the upper limits of normal, as in LVH, but it cannot be 0.10 s or greater. Nevertheless, a pattern of incomplete RBBB can sometimes be seen with RVH, but cannot be used to reliably diagnose RVH.

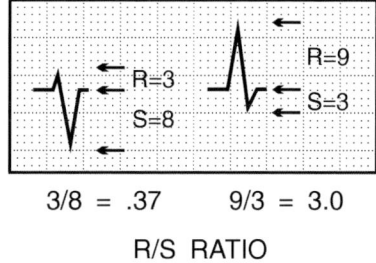

$$3/8 = .37 \qquad 9/3 = 3.0$$

R/S RATIO

Figure 8.4. Calculation of the R-to-S ratio in any lead.

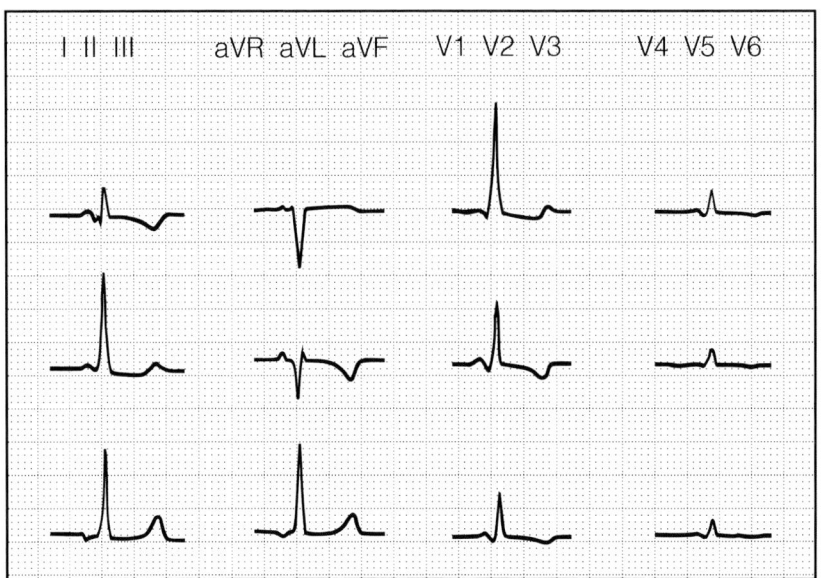

Figure 8.5. Fully developed RVH with a strain pattern in the leads that look at the right ventricle, namely the right-sided precordial leads. This tracing is from a 12-year-old female with congenital heart disease and a single right ventricle.

The fully developed strain pattern of RVH, like that of LVH, consists of an upwardly convex ST depression blending into an inverted T wave, but now is seen in the right precordial leads (V_1 and V_2), which, of course, look at the right ventricle (Figure 8.5). The strain pattern may also frequently be seen in those limb leads toward which the main vector of ventricular depolarization is headed (electrical axis). In RVH, this is frequently lead aVF or III because of RAD.

Summary of Criteria for RVH

Remember, again, that the electrocardiographic criteria for chamber enlargement have both low sensitivity and specificity. In summary, these are the things to look for when trying to diagnose RVH:

1. R to S ratio of >1.0 in V_1 or V_2
2. RAD
3. Normal QRS duration
4. Strain pattern V_1 or V_2 and in limb leads with the tallest R wave

Practice Tracings

Answers to the practice tracings (Figures 8.6 and 8.7) on the following pages may be found in the Chapter 14.

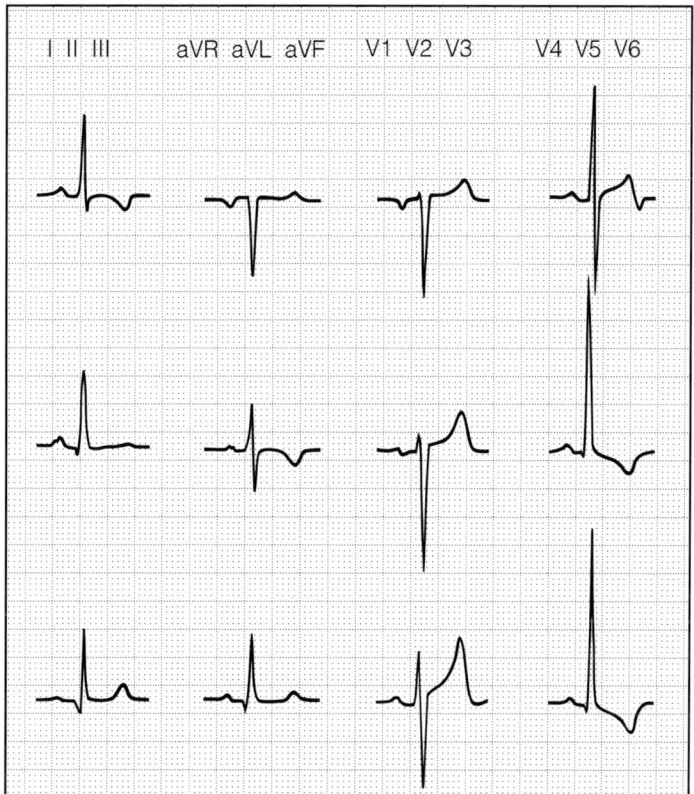

Figure 8.6. Practice tracing.

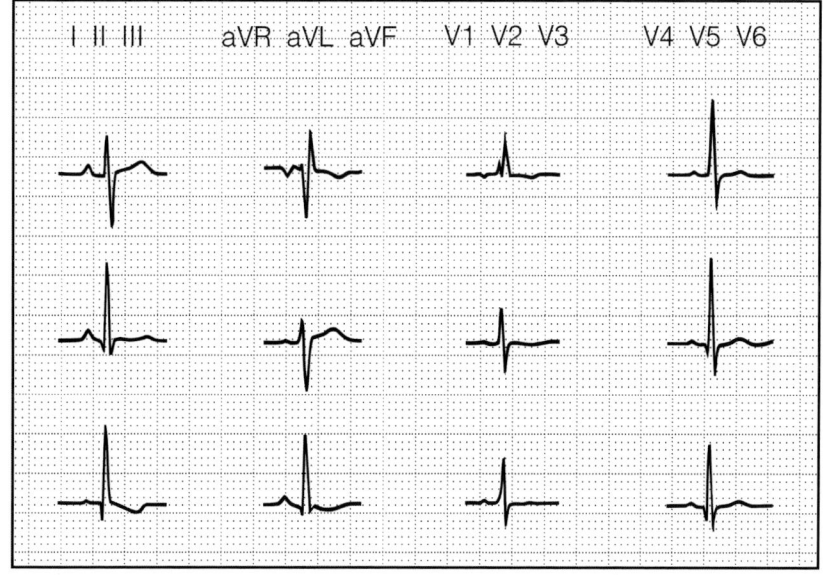

Figure 8.7. Practice tracing.

9

Myocardial Infarction

In this chapter, we will discuss what is, for ACLS providers, perhaps the most important and certainly the most clinically interesting subject in 12-lead electrocardiography: AMI.

Anatomy of the Coronary Arteries

The coronary arterial circulation begins with the divergence of the right and left coronary arteries from the aorta. The *left main coronary artery* is very short and rapidly splits into the *left anterior descending artery* and the *circumflex artery*.

The right coronary artery serves primarily the *right ventricle* and the *inferior* and *true posterior* walls of the left ventricle. The right coronary artery also gives off the *AV nodal artery* in approximately 90% of patients. The left anterior descending artery serves the *anterior wall* of the left ventricle, and the circumflex artery serves the *left lateral wall* of the left ventricle. Figure 9.1 illustrates these relationships.

Pathophysiology of AMI

Acute myocardial infarction occurs any time that a coronary artery becomes essentially completely obstructed and the segment of myocardium served by that artery loses perfusion and begins to die.

Complete obstruction usually occurs in the setting of *fixed obstructive coronary lesions* that are the result of coronary atherosclerosis. However, the process of accumulating *atherosclerotic plaque* in the coronary arteries is slow and gradual. The acute nature of AMI is usually the result of a clot or *thrombus* forming in the immediate vicinity of an incomplete fixed obstructive lesion.

The cause of clot formation is typically *rupture* (a split) of an atherosclerotic plaque, which tears the overlying endothelium thereby exposing blood to the lipid-rich interior of the plaque. Many of the substances present in the

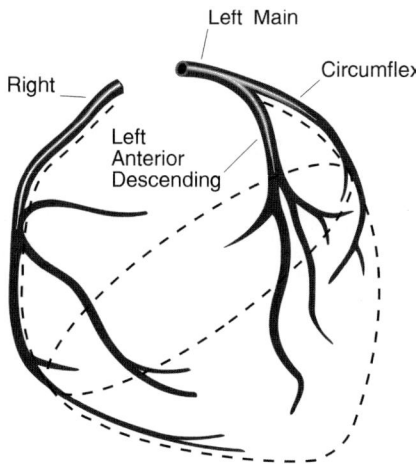

Figure 9.1. The coronary arterial circulation.

plaque interior stimulate both platelet aggregation and the coagulation cascade, resulting in thrombus formation.

Less than complete obstruction of the coronary arteries can produce *ischemia* (diminished perfusion) without actual death of tissue, and is the cause of the syndrome called *angina*.

Electrocardiographic Categories of AMI

There are two electrocardiographic categories of AMI, which are based on whether or not the infarction produces ST segment elevation on the electrocardiogram. The first category is called ST-segment elevation myocardial infarction (*STEMI*).

The second category of infarction does not produce ST-segment elevation and is called a non-STEMI (*NSTEMI*). You will learn in a subsequent chapter that these two categories have great practical clinical significance because the treatment for the two categories is so different.

We will consider the electrocardiographic hallmarks of STEMI first because it produces the classic ECG changes of ST-segment elevation that many people recognize as being associated with AMI.

Electrocardiographic Hallmarks of STEMI

Figure 9.2 illustrates the following three ECG hallmarks of a classic STEMI:

1. ST-segment elevation
2. T wave inversion
3. Q wave formation

These three changes in the ECG typically *evolve* over a period of minutes to hours, with ST elevation usually appearing first, followed variably by T wave inversion and Q wave formation. Subsequently, the changes may show slow resolution, usually over a period ranging from days to months. Q waves, however, may persist indefinitely, producing ECG evidence of a *scar*.

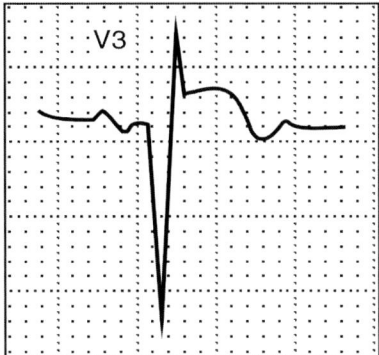

Figure 9.2. The three ECG hallmarks of AMI, including ST elevation, T wave inversion, and Q wave formation.

This sequence of changes is called *electrocardiographic evolution* of an infarction (Figure 9.3). It is important to recognize that the ECG diagnosis of AMI is much more accurate when made on the basis of evolution over a series of tracings than when made on the basis of a single ECG. Keep in mind also that the ECG may not reveal clear patterns of infarction in the earliest stages of evolution.

On occasion, the earliest change of AMI, occurring even before ST segment elevation, may actually be an increase in the height of the T wave called

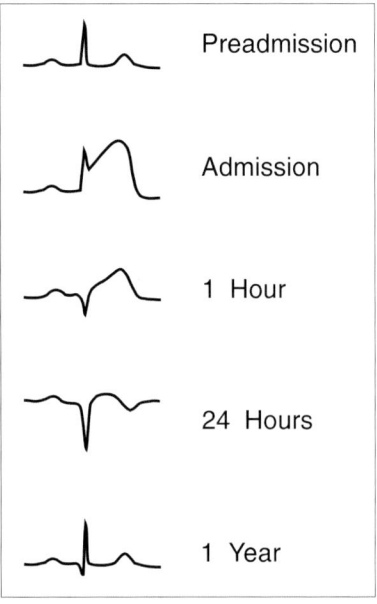

Figure 9.3. The evolution of an inferior wall myocardial infarction, as seen in lead III of a 55-year-old white male. Note that the admission tracing shows only ST elevation. A Q wave is beginning to form by 1 hour, and ST elevation is on the way down. By 24 hours, Q wave formation is complete, and the T wave is fully inverted. By 1 year, a pathologic Q wave is the only remaining evidence of infarction.

hyperacute T wave changes. Hyperacute T waves alone are insufficient evidence with which to make the diagnosis of AMI. When seen, however, they should increase your index of suspicion for AMI in a patient presenting with signs and symptoms that are compatible with AMI.

You may have deduced from this discussion that it is extremely important to correlate clinical signs and symptoms with the ECG before making the diagnosis of AMI. More on that later.

Localization of Infarction

It is often possible to determine in a general way which wall of the heart is involved in a STEMI by determining in which leads we see the three hallmarks of STEMI.

You will recall from Chapter 3 and from your knowledge of the hexaxial reference system (Figure 9.4) that leads II, III, and aVF are called the inferior leads because they look up at the heart from below. When the typical evolution of the three hallmarks of STEMI is seen in II, III, and aVF, we label it an *inferior wall myocardial infarction.*

If the ST elevation, T wave inversion, and Q wave formation are seen in leads I and aVL, we call it a *lateral wall infarction* because leads I and aVL look at the lateral wall of the heart.

Finally, if we see evolutionary changes across V_2–V_4, we label it *anterior wall infarction* because the precordial leads look at the anterior wall of the heart. When lead V_1 is also involved it is sometimes called an *anteroseptal infarction.*

Either inferior or anterior wall infarctions can also sometimes show changes in the far lateral precordial leads (V_5 and V_6) as well as in leads I and aVL. The descriptive terms *inferolateral* or *anterolateral* are then used to locate the infarction.

Electrocardiographers usually require that the changes of STEMI be seen in two or more *contiguous leads* (adjacent leads) on the hexaxial reference

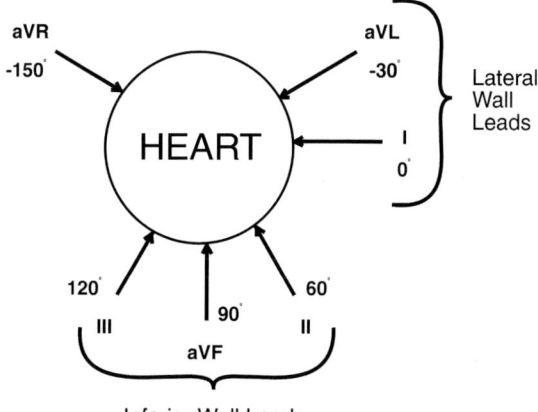

Figure 9.4. The hexaxial reference system showing those leads that are considered to reflect the inferior and lateral walls of the heart.

system or among the precordial leads before a diagnosis of infarction is made. For example, to diagnose an inferior STEMI, one would have to see changes in at least leads II and aVF, or in leads aVF and III, because each of these pairs of leads are contiguous.

ST Elevation

ST elevation in AMI occurs in the presence of myocardium that is in the process of dying, and it is often called a *current of injury*. It typically appears in those infarctions that are *transmural*, meaning they involve the full

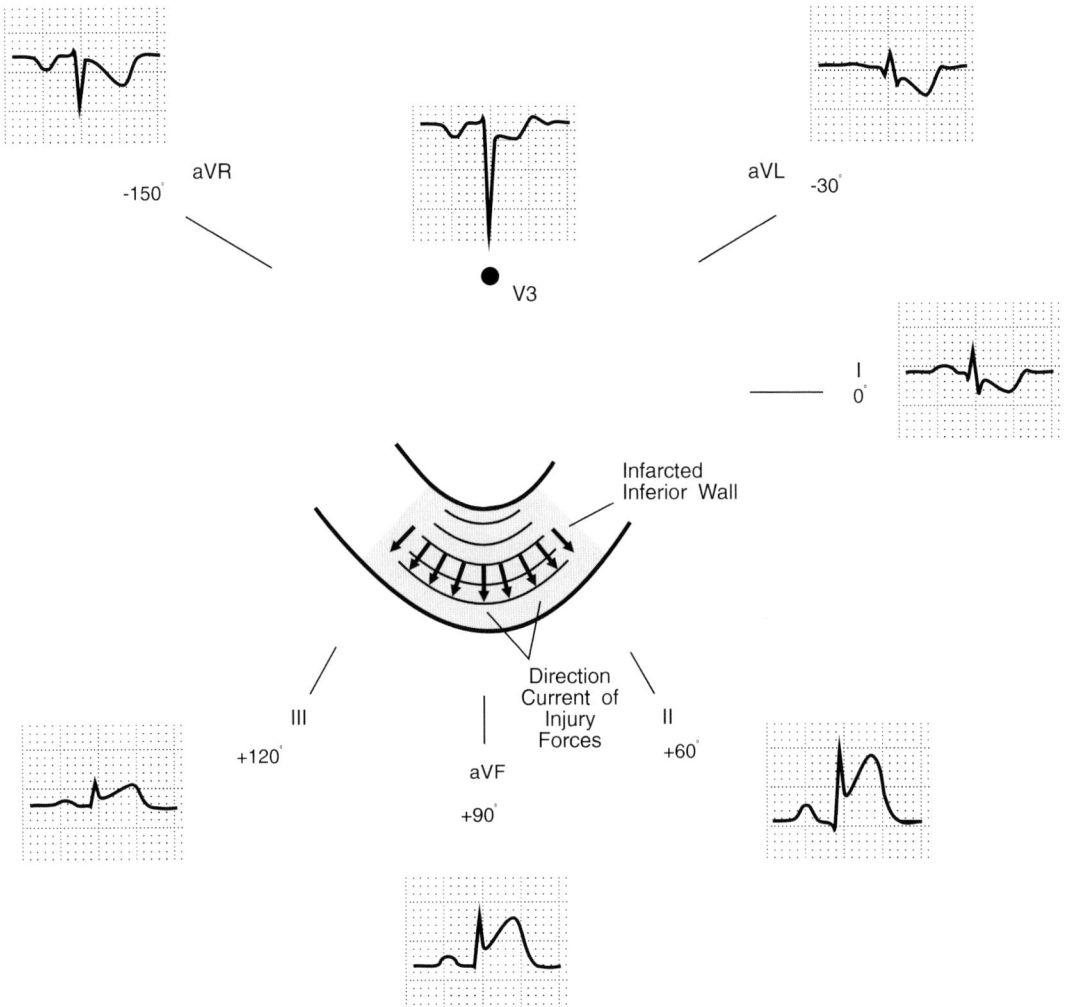

Figure 9.5. Inferior wall AMI producing ST elevation in leads II, III, and aVF. Note that while the force vectors of the current of injury are coming toward II, III, and aVF, they are going away from the reciprocal leads of I and aVL, and the precordial leads represented in the diagram by V₃. The deviation of the ECG needle is therefore negative in the reciprocal leads, producing what is called reciprocal ST depression.

thickness of the ventricular wall as opposed to a partial thickness. Most STEMIs are therefore transmural.

Note in Figure 9.2 that the ST elevation of AMI is typically, but not always, *upwardly convex*, meaning that it bows upward. This produces an appearance that some have likened to that of a fireman's cap. However, ST elevation may also be upwardly concave.

Because ST elevation is an upward deflection of the ECG needle, it is clear that the current of injury in the infarcted wall of myocardium is producing force vectors similar to those of a T wave that are coming toward the lead in which we view the ST elevation. In other words, the current of injury is spreading from endocardium to epicardium.

In Figure 9.5, we see the force vectors of a current of injury in the inferior wall coming toward leads II, III, and aVF and producing ST elevation in those leads. By the same token, the force vectors are going away from the leads in the *reciprocal* or opposite leads I and aVL and the precordial leads of V_2–V_2, represented in the diagram by V_3. This produces what is called *reciprocal depression* in the wall of the heart opposite the location of the infarction.

Thus, inferior wall STEMIs produce reciprocal depression in the anterior and high lateral walls (leads V_2–V_4 and I and aVL). Anterior STEMIs produce reciprocal depression in the inferior wall (leads II, III, and aVF), as shown in Figure 9.6.

However, classical reciprocal depression does not always appear with the ST elevation of AMI. Reciprocal depression is fleeting, and depending on the timing of the tracing, a substantial number of acute infarctions may not show it. When present, however, reciprocal depression greatly enhances the confidence of labeling an infarction as acute (as opposed to old).

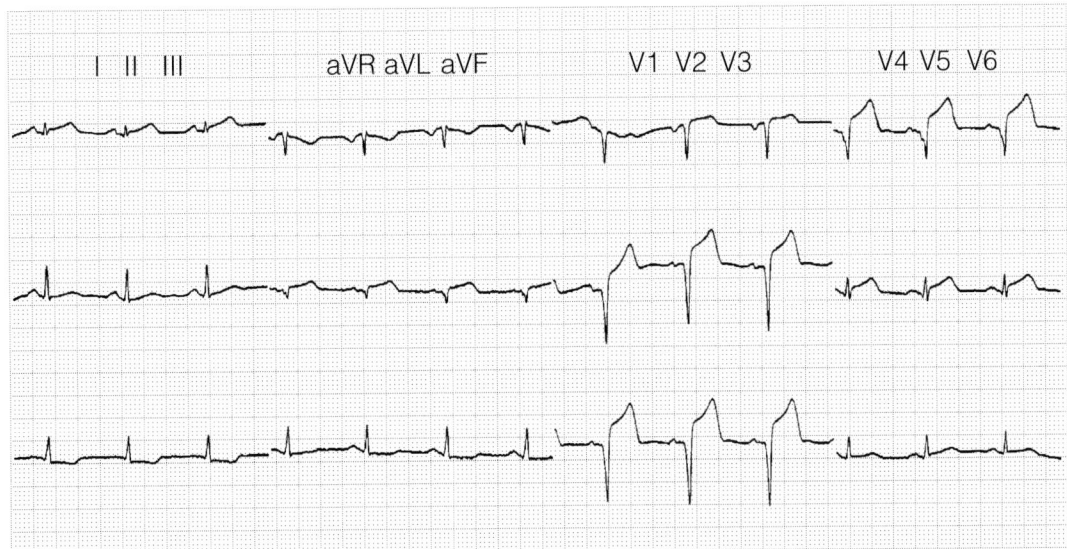

Figure 9.6. Acute anterior wall myocardial infarction. Note that, in addition to ST-segment elevation across the anterior precordial leads, there is reciprocal depression seen in leads III and aVF. Also note that, in this particular patient, the ST elevation is slightly upwardly concave.

When ST elevation alone is seen without other confirming evidence of AMI, most electrocardiographers require for diagnosis that at least 1 mm of elevation be seen in two or more contiguous limb leads for inferior infarctions and at least 2 mm in two or more contiguous precordial leads for anterior wall infarctions.

Other Causes of ST Segment Elevation

ST elevation itself is not confined exclusively to STEMI. Other conditions can cause ST elevation, including pericarditis and ventricular aneurysm. ST elevation can even be seen as a normal variant in healthy people. There are ways, however, to differentiate these other causes of ST elevation from AMI. These methods will be discussed later in this chapter under Differential Diagnosis of ST Elevation.

T Wave Inversion

As the ST elevation seen in STEMI begins to come down, the T wave also begins to come down from its upright position, and eventually inverts. In the intermediate position, it is frequently biphasic. Figure 9.7 shows an anterolateral wall STEMI, substantially far along in evolution, with slight remaining ST elevation and prominent T wave inversion in V_2–V_5 and I and aVL.

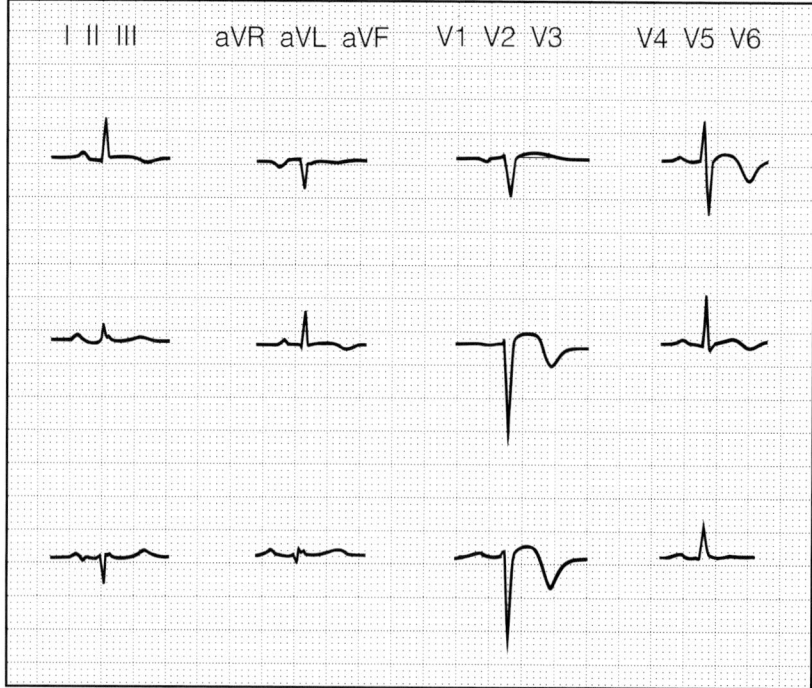

Figure 9.7. Evolving anterior wall myocardial infarction showing loss of R wave progression in V_2–V_4. Slight ST elevation remains, and there is prominent T wave inversion in leads V_2–V_5, I, and aVL.

Q Wave Formation

When a transmural segment of myocardium undergoes infarction, it ceases to depolarize normally and becomes essentially *electrically inert*. As a result, there are no forces of ventricular depolarization spreading from endocardium to epicardium and coming directly toward whichever leads are viewing the infarcted wall. Instead, the leads viewing the infarction are looking through the "window" of inactive infarcted myocardium at the forces of the opposite wall of the ventricle. These vectors in the opposite wall are also spreading from endocardium to epicardium and are therefore going away from the leads looking at the infarction. This concept of an *electrical window* through the infarction looking on the "back wall" of the heart, as illustrated in Figure 9.8, is a simplified but useful concept for explaining Q wave formation in the leads looking at the infarction.

In an anterior wall infarction, for example, as the anterior wall begins to die, the forces of anterior wall depolarization spreading from endocardium to epicardium gradually decline until they cease. As a result, the R wave normally seen in the anterior precordial leads gradually becomes smaller and smaller until the initial deflection finally becomes a Q. This is called *loss of R wave progression* across the precordium. Figure 9.7 shows substantial loss of the normal R wave in V_2–V_4, but actual Q wave formation has not yet occurred. Figure 9.6 shows full Q wave formation in leads V_1–V_5.

You will recall from our previous discussion of the normal ECG that, as a result of left-to-right septal depolarization, a small Q wave can be

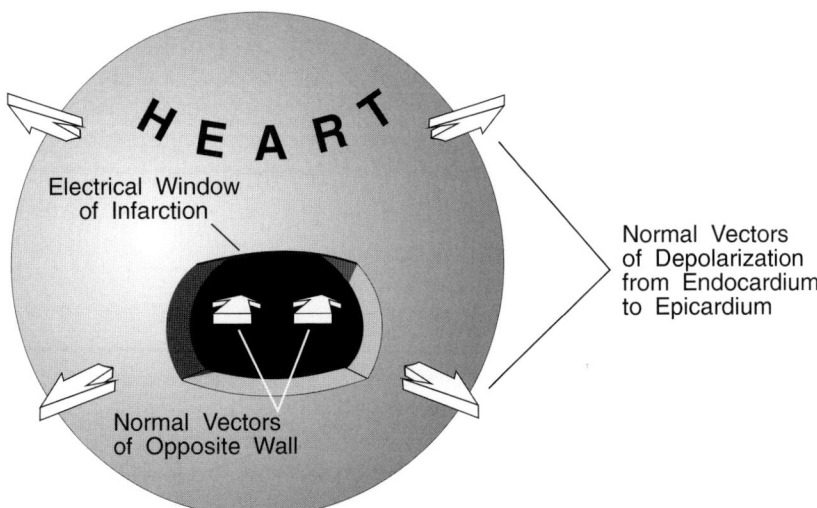

Figure 9.8. Q wave formation in AMI. Schematic diagram of the heart illustrating how the "window" of electrically inert infarcted tissue in AMI permits the electrode viewing the infarction to look through the window at the opposite wall of the heart. Normal force vectors in the opposite wall are going away from the electrode, traveling from endocardium to epicardium, producing a negative deflection that we call a Q wave.

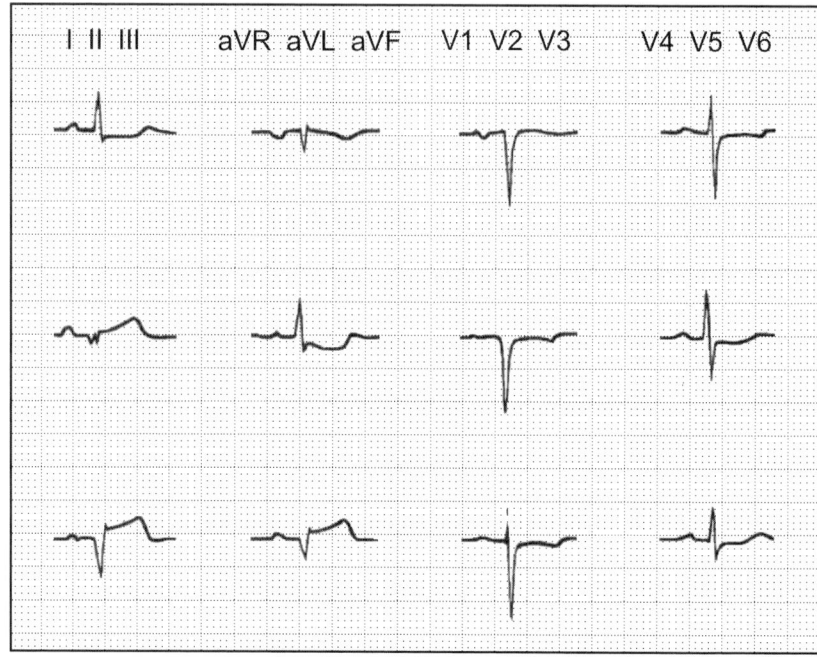

Figure 9.9. Acute inferior wall myocardial infarction showing pathologic Q wave formation and ST elevation in II, III, and aVF. A pathologic Q wave can also be seen in leads V_1 and V_2, denoting an old anterior wall infarction.

normally seen in the inferior leads II and aVF particularly. Q waves will also be seen in lead III with LPH. With acute inferior wall infarction, however, the Q becomes deeper and wider until it reaches criteria for becoming what electrocardiographers call a *pathologic Q wave*. Most electrocardiographers define a pathologic Q as being at least 0.04 s wide (one small block) with a depth > 25% of the height of the R wave. Thus, the presence of a Q wave alone in the inferior leads is not enough to diagnose an inferior wall infarction, unless the Q wave is pathologic. Figure 9.9 shows an acute inferior wall myocardial infarction with pathologic Q wave formation along with ST elevation in leads II, III, and aVF.

Q Waves as Scars

It was mentioned earlier in the chapter that the ST elevation and T wave inversion seen in STEMI frequently resolve over time, but that the Q wave may persist indefinitely as evidence of a past infarction. Pathologic Q waves in the absence of AMI are therefore sometimes referred to in ECG reports as *scars* or *remote infarctions*. Figures 9.10 and 9.11 show remote inferior and anterior infarctions, respectively, in which the ST elevation and T wave inversion have resolved but Q waves persist as evidence of the old infarction. Close inspection of the acute inferior myocardial infarction shown in Figure 9.9 also reveals a pathologic Q wave in V_1 and V_2, indicating an old anteroseptal wall infarction.

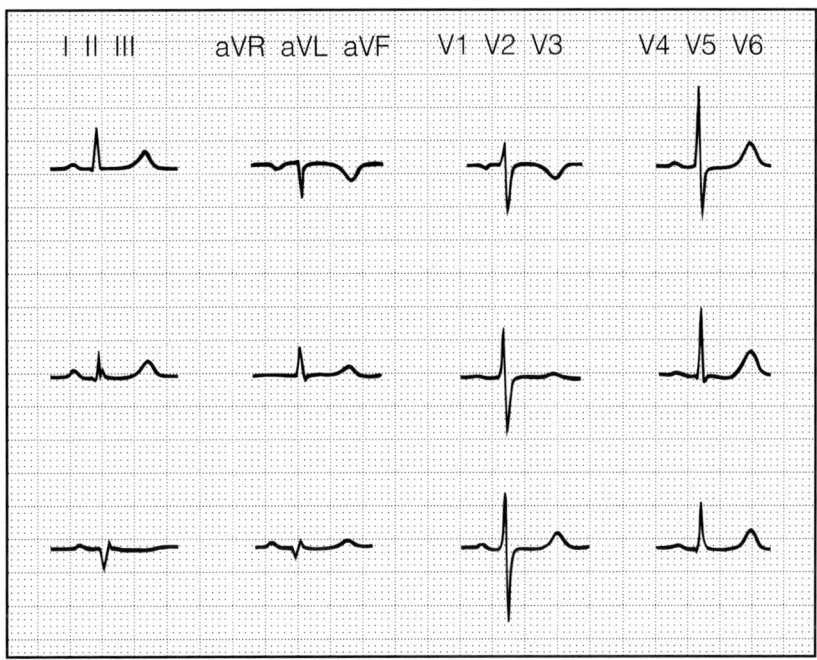

Figure 9.10. Remote inferior wall myocardial infarction showing pathologic Q wave formation in leads III and aVF.

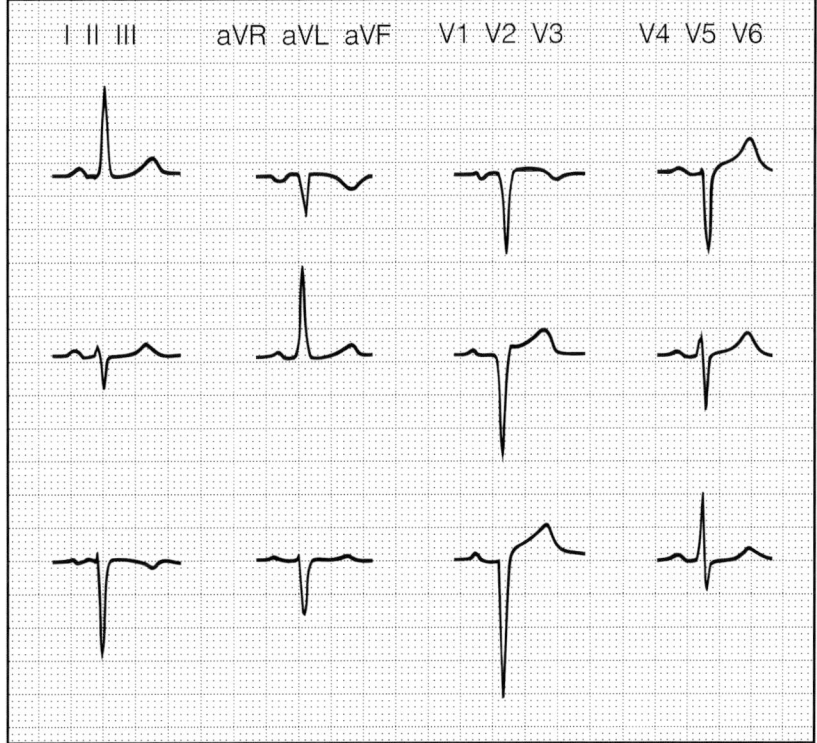

Figure 9.11. Remote anterior wall myocardial infarction showing pathologic Q wave formation in V_1–V_3. Although there is still slight ST elevation that has persisted, as is sometimes the case with large infarctions, note that there is no reciprocal depression in the inferior leads and that T waves are upright in leads V_2–V_6

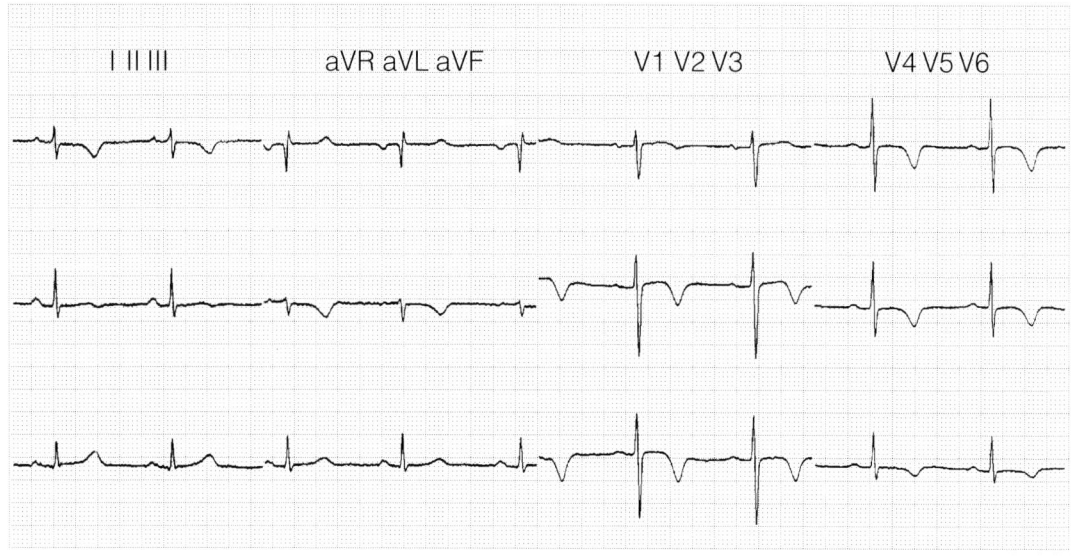

Figure 9.12. Non–Q wave infarction of the anterior wall. Note the deep T wave inversion across the precordium and the absence of Q waves.

Non–Q Wave Infarctions

Sometimes in AMI, if the infarction is small or if it does not involve the full thickness of the myocardial wall, an actual Q wave will never develop. This is called a *non–Q wave infarction.*

In anterior wall non–Q wave infarctions, we may see loss of R wave progression, even though the Q never forms. With inferior wall non–Q wave infarctions, either a Q never forms or the normal Q wave, if present, simply never becomes deep enough or wide enough to meet criteria for a pathologic Q wave.

Non–Q wave infarctions, therefore, must be diagnosed electrocardiographically solely on the basis of evolution in the ST segment and T wave. Figure 9.12 shows a non–Q wave infarction of the anterior wall with deep T wave inversion across the precordium but no loss of R wave. There is still a hint of ST segment elevation present.

Non-ST Segment Elevation Myocardial Infarction

Only approximately one third of patients with non–Q wave infarctions ever develop ST elevation. The remaining two thirds develop ST depression alone, variably followed by T wave inversion. This group of patients falls into the category of NSTEMI.

This frustrating category of AMI presents an enormous diagnostic challenge to every clinician because it is often impossible electrocardiographically to distinguish patients with NSTEMI from those with the syndrome of unstable angina without infarction. It is often only when biochemical cardiac markers (cardiac enzymes) begin to rise that one is able to make a clear diagnosis of NSTEMI. You will learn more about unstable angina and the electrocardiographic features of ischemia in the next chapter.

Indeed, some patients who are undergoing a NSTEMI may present with a perfectly normal ECG initially, and even with the passage of time demonstrate only subtle ST and T wave changes.

Figure 9.13 is the tracing of a 48-year-old white male who presented in the early morning hours with retrosternal pain that he described as feeling like his usual pain of esophageal reflux, but slightly more intense and lasting longer. By now you have the skills to conclude that his initial ECG was, indeed, perfectly normal.

By midmorning, however, he had developed elevated cardiac enzymes, and it was not until 4 hours after his initial ECG that he began to display some ST and T wave changes in the anterior wall that supported the evolution of an NSTEMI, as seen in Figure 9.14.

As you have undoubtedly surmised, this is a treacherous diagnostic category. Clinicians must maintain a high index of suspicion, as well as rely on the full spectrum of diagnostic modalities, in order not to miss this often difficult, but potentially lethal, diagnosis.

This patient provides us with our first hard lesson that one must always correlate the ECG with the history, physical examination, and other pertinent data, rather than relying on the ECG alone for diagnosis. More on that in a subsequent chapter.

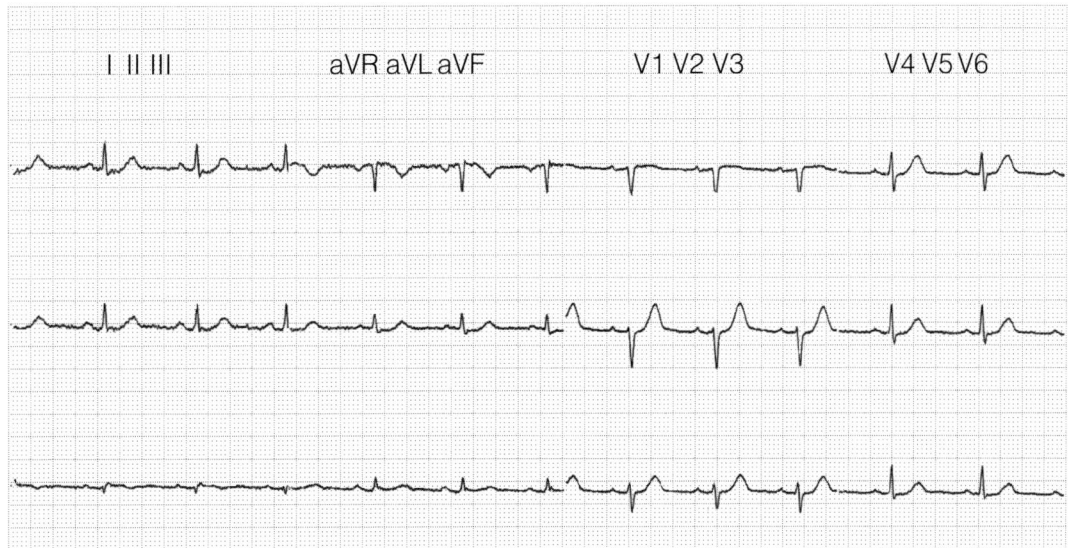

Figure 9.13. Presenting ECG of a patient with NSTEMI. Note the absence of any clear indication of an acute coronary syndrome on this ECG.

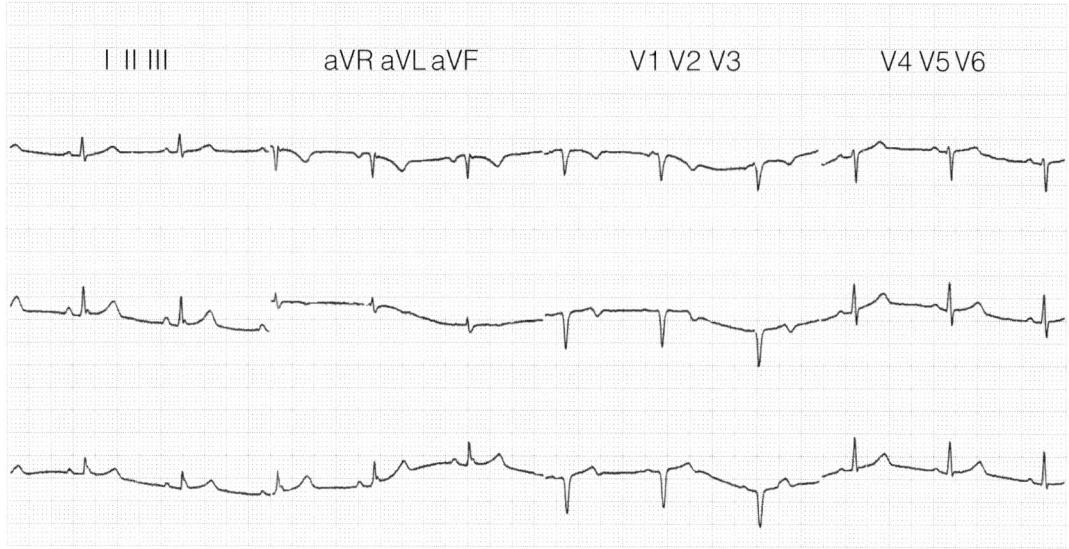

Figure 9.14. ECG of patient in Figure 9.13, 4 hours later. By 4 hours after the initial ECG shown in Figure 9.13, this patient had positive biomarkers for infarction, and was developing loss of R wave across the precordium, with T wave inversion.

Differential Diagnosis of ST Elevation

Acute myocardial infarction is not the only condition that can cause ST-segment elevation. Several other conditions, including *pericarditis* and *benign early repolarization changes* (a normal variant of ST elevation commonly seen in healthy young adults), routinely produce ST elevation. It is important, therefore, to distinguish STEMI from other causes of ST elevation.

Several distinguishing criteria can be helpful. First, as described earlier in this chapter, the ST elevation of AMI is often accompanied by reciprocal depression in the wall opposite the infarction. Pericarditis and benign early repolarization changes, however, show no reciprocal depression but, instead, show ST elevation in all walls. In other words, the ST elevation is not localized to one wall, but is widespread and is reflected in more than one ECG region of the heart.

Figure 9.15 shows the tracing of a young adult male with acute pericarditis. Note that the ST elevation is widespread throughout the inferior, anterior, and lateral walls, and that there is no reciprocal depression. Another very helpful clue that this tracing represents pericarditis rather than STEMI is the presence of *PR-segment depression*. Note that the PR segment shows slightly downsloping depression in all leads. This finding is characteristic of pericarditis.

Figure 9.16 is the tracing of a healthy, asymptomatic 34-year-old male who has no clinical evidence of pericardial or myocardial disease. This tracing is typical of benign early repolarization changes and, like pericarditis, shows widespread ST elevation without reciprocal depression. Unlike pericarditis, however, there is no PR-segment depression.

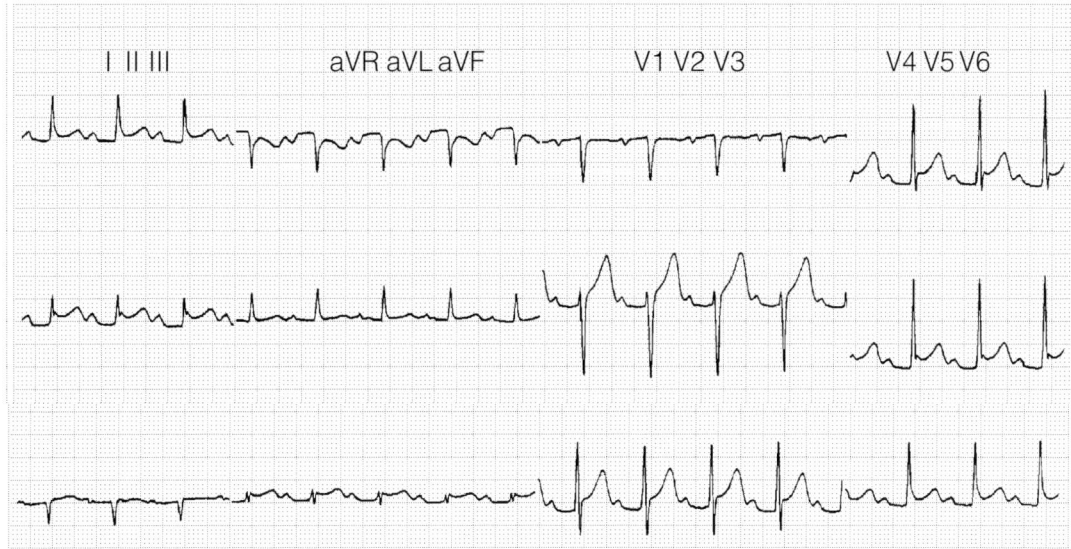

Figure 9.15. Acute pericarditis. Note that there is widespread ST elevation that is upwardly deeply concave in the anterior, inferior, and lateral walls. In addition, there is no reciprocal depression and there are no Q waves.

A second helpful distinguishing criterion between AMI and these other two causes of ST elevation is that the ST-segment elevation of AMI is typically upwardly convex or only very slightly concave. Note in Figures 9.15 and 9.16, however, that the ST elevation of pericarditis and benign early repolarization changes is typically *downwardly convex*.

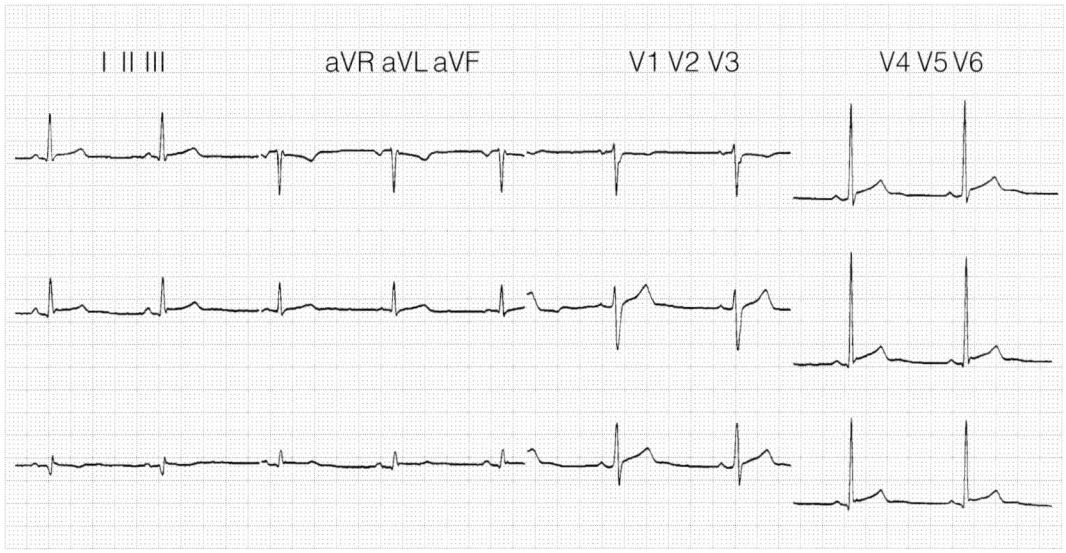

Figure 9.16. Benign early repolarization changes. Note that, as in pericarditis, there is widespread ST elevation that is upwardly concave, although it is usually not as high as in pericarditis. In addition, there is no reciprocal depression, and there are no Q waves or T wave inversions.

Difficult to Diagnose Infarctions

Right Ventricular AMI

Most infarctions involve the left ventricle, sparing the right ventricle. As you have learned, the right ventricle is supplied by the right coronary artery. When a very proximal right coronary artery occlusion occurs, not only will infarction occur in the inferior wall of the left ventricle, but as many as 50% of these patients may also have some involvement of the right ventricle as well. However, placement of the leads in the standard 12-lead electrocardiogram provides views primarily only of the left ventricle.

To see infarction of the right ventricle, it may be necessary to place V leads on the right side of the chest in positions corresponding to those used routinely on the left side of the chest. These leads are called $V_1R–V_6R$.

True Posterior AMI

The right coronary artery also supplies the true posterior wall of the left ventricle. Thus, occlusions of the right coronary artery may not only produce the familiar pattern of inferior wall infarction but may also produce an infarction of the true posterior wall that is more difficult to diagnose in the standard 12-lead ECG.

Because the endocardium-to-epicardium force vectors of the current of injury in infarction of the true posterior wall are going away from our precordial electrodes, infarction of the true posterior wall produces a mirror image of anterior wall infarctions. That is, one may see very tall R waves in leads $V_1–V_3$ corresponding to Q waves in the posterior wall, as well as deep ST depression and T wave inversion in leads $V_1–V_3$ corresponding to ST elevation and hyperacute T waves of the true posterior wall infarction in progress. In other words, when looking at the changes of a true posterior infarction in the V leads of the precordium, we are really seeing reciprocal ST depression from the posterior wall ST-segment elevation.

Thus, seeing a tall R wave with an R-to-S ratio > 1.0 in $V_1–V_3$ coupled with deep ST-segment depression and T wave inversion in a patient presenting with symptoms compatible with AMI should raise the suspicion of a true posterior AMI. This suspicion can be confirmed by placing leads on the posterior chest in a position horizontal to lead V_6 (called $V_7–V_9$), or by seeing posterior wall motion abnormalities on an echocardiogram that are consistent with a true posterior infarction.

Other Pitfalls to Diagnosing AMI

Ventricular Aneurysm

Earlier in this chapter, it was mentioned that observing the evolution of AMI on serial ECG tracings leads to a more accurate diagnosis than does reading a single tracing. One of the reasons why this is true is that, occasionally,

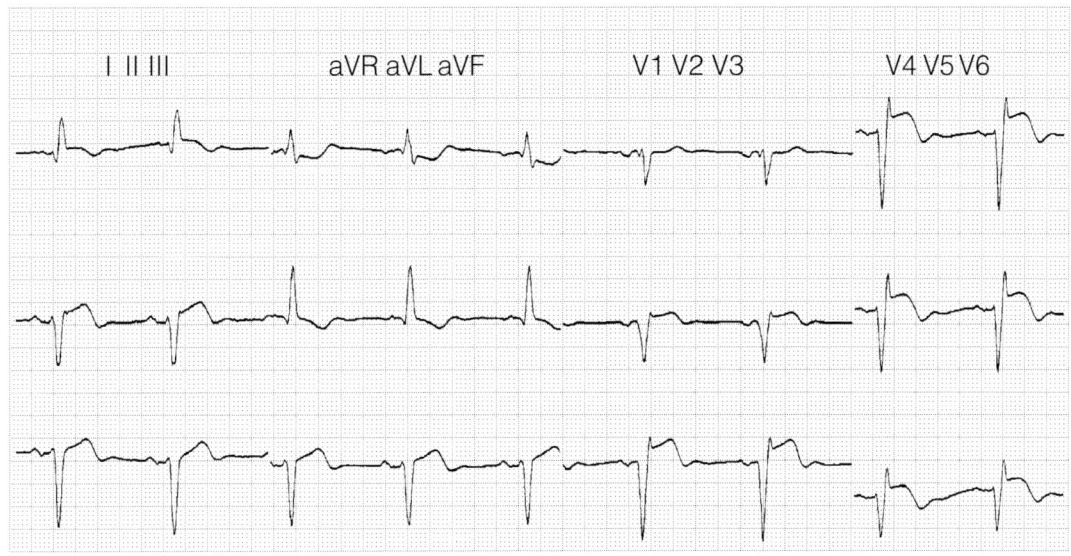

Figure 9.17. Ventricular aneurysm. Persistent ST elevation 4 years after acute anterior wall infarction in a 75-year-old male with aneurysm of the left ventricle proven by echocardiogram. Note the absence of reciprocal depression as one of the clues that this infarction may be old.

ST-segment elevation may persist for many months after STEMI. This is particularly true of large anterior infarctions. Indeed, the electrocardiographic diagnosis of a *ventricular aneurysm* is based upon *ST elevation persisting indefinitely* after AMI (Figure 9.17). Therefore, it is easy to mistakenly conclude on the basis of a single, random ECG that a patient with a ventricular aneurysm is in the process of having an AMI, when in actuality the infarction may be months or years old.

If the aneurysm is very large, as in the patient whose ECG is shown in Figure 9.17, the ST elevation may even extend into the lateral and inferior walls.

A clue to the age of the infarction shown in Figure 9.17, however, is that there is no reciprocal depression. The absence of reciprocal depression is characteristic of old infarctions that demonstrate persistent ST elevation. When there is a question of whether an ECG infarction pattern is new or old, the presence of reciprocal depression lends strong support to the conclusion that the infarction is acute. Conversely, the absence of reciprocal depression should raise the question in the reader's mind of whether observed ST elevation may actually represent ventricular aneurysm as the result of a remote infarction. The best way to deal with the question of age is to always compare the current tracing with a previous one on file and to lay heavy emphasis on correlation of the current ECG with the clinical picture.

Left Bundle Branch Block

Another potential pitfall to the diagnosis of AMI lies in patients with LBBB. As shown in Figure 9.18, and as you already know, LBBB often

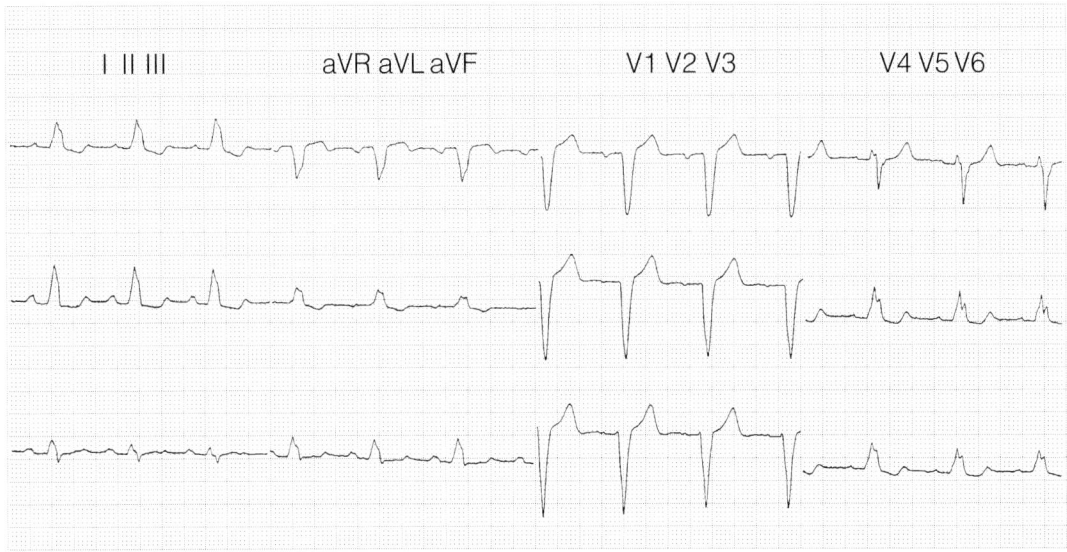

Figure 9.18. Left bundle branch block simulating anterior wall infarction. Q waves in V₂ and V₃, together with upward slurring of the ST segments, can often be mistaken for acute anterior wall infarction if one does not notice that the QRS duration is 0.12 s or greater and that there is an RSR′ in the lateral precordial leads.

produces Q waves in the anterior precordial leads, along with upward slurring of the ST segment. This combination can simulate the ST segment elevation of acute anterior wall infarction. But the converse is also true. Some patients with extensive anterior wall infarctions develop LBBB because of extensive necrosis of the septum. Indeed, diagnosing anterior wall myocardial infarction in patients with LBBB is so perilous that the safest course for all but the most experienced electrocardio-graphers is to never try to make an electrocardiographic diagnosis of anterior wall myocardial infarction in patients with LBBB. In this situation, the clinical presentation becomes all-important, as we will discuss in Chapter 11. The availability of an old tracing on file is also of paramount importance, so that one may establish whether or not the LBBB is new.

That being said, there are some clues that can be used to detect anterior AMI in a patient with LBBB. Figure 9.19 shows a tracing with a QRS duration of 0.12 s and a LBBB pattern. Note, however, the difference in the anterior wall ST segments and T waves between this tracing and the tracing in Figure 9.18. In Figure 9.18 the T waves in lead V₂ are inscribed in the opposite direction of the main deflection of the QRS, as is usually the case in BBB. However, in Figure 9.19 you will note that the T waves in lead V₂ are *concordant*, meaning that they are inscribed in the same direction as the main deflection of the QRS. These changes may suggest an evolving anterior AMI.

Because the pattern of LBBB in the inferior leads does not produce giant Q waves, it is easier to diagnose inferior wall AMI in patients with LBBB.

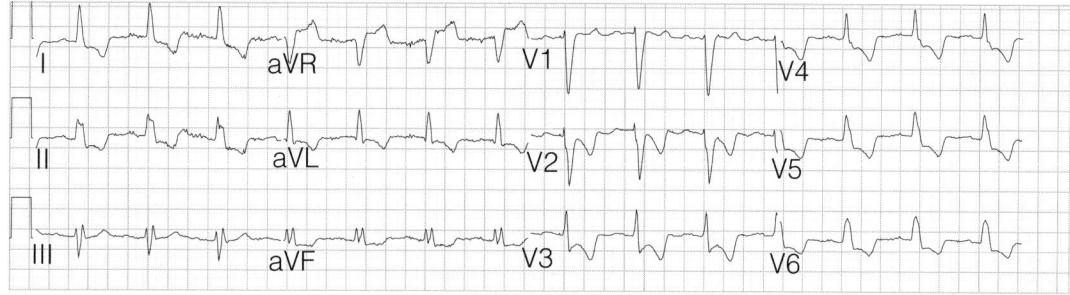

Figure 9.19. Evolving anterior wall myocardial infarction in the presence of LBBB. Note that the T waves in lead V$_2$ are concordant, meaning that they are inscribed in the same direction as the QRS. This is in contrast to the T waves in the anterior wall in Figure 9.19, which are discordant, meaning that they are inscribed in the opposite direction of the QRS, as is normally the case in LBBB.

Right Bundle Branch Block

Unlike LBBB, however, it is often possible to make the diagnosis of acute STEMI in patients with RBBB.

Figure 9.20 shows the tracing of a 52-year-old white male who presented with typical clinical symptoms of AMI. Although having a QRS duration >0.12 s and having the typical RSR' in lead V$_1$ of RBBB, note that one can still clearly see ST-segment elevation in leads III and aVF, and that reciprocal depression is visible in leads V$_2$ and V$_3$.

Left Anterior Hemiblock

A final pitfall worthy of consideration is the presence of LAH, as discussed at length in Chapter 6. Figures 6.6 and 6.7 demonstrate that the extreme LAD of LAH can simulate the Q waves of remote inferior wall infarction if one does not search carefully for the tiny R waves in leads II, III, and aVF that are part of the criteria for LAH.

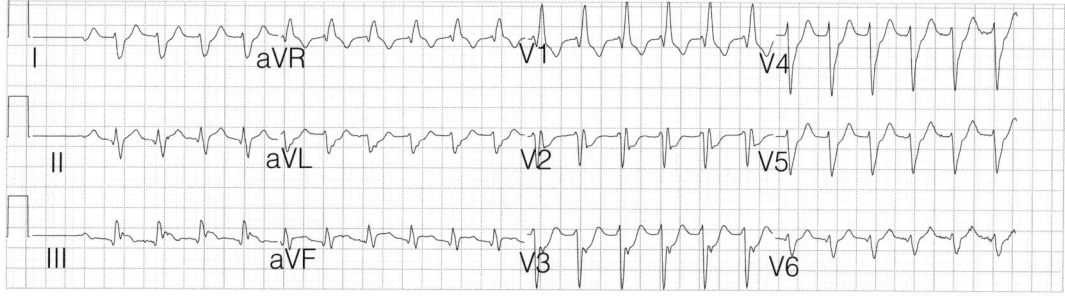

Figure 9.20. Acute inferior wall STEMI in the presence of RBBB. ST elevation can still be seen in leads II, III, and aVF despite RBBB, as well as J point depression (reciprocal depression) in the anterior wall and leads I and aVL.

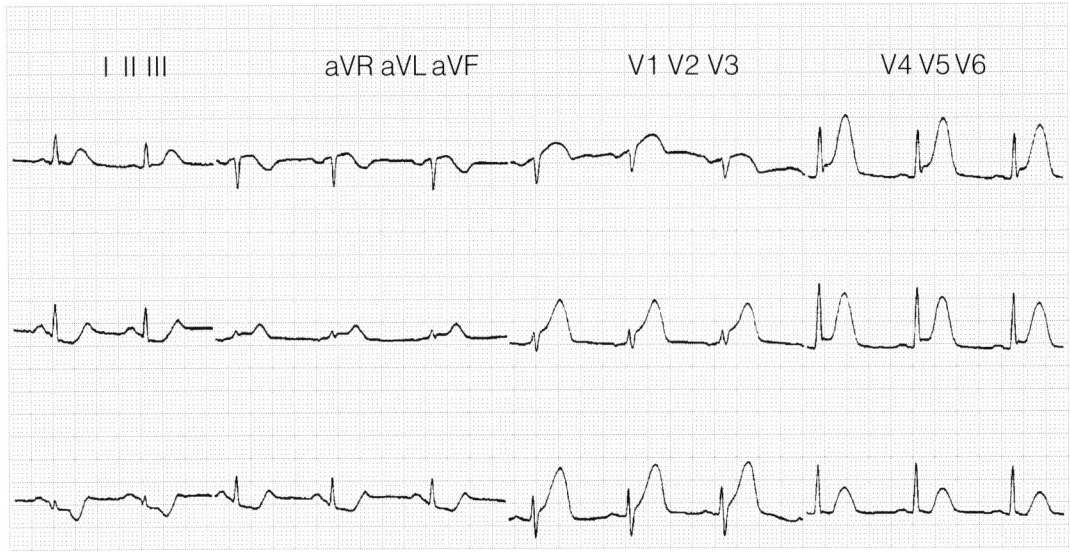

Figure 9.21. Practice tracing.

Practice Tracings

The tracings in Figures 9.21 to 9.25 are for practicing your new skills at diagnosing myocardial infarction. The answers may be found at the end of Chapter 14.

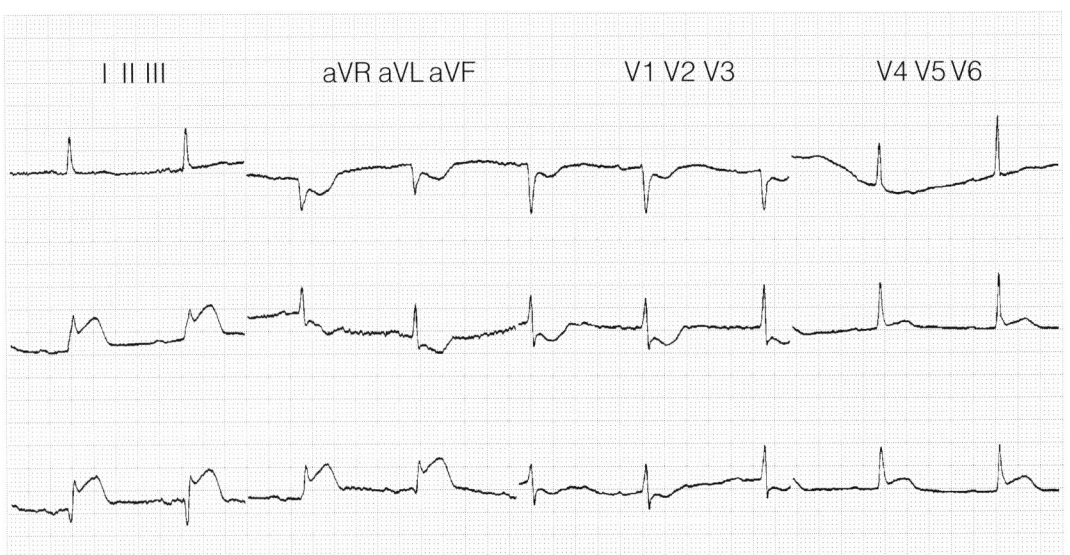

Figure 9.22. Practice tracing.

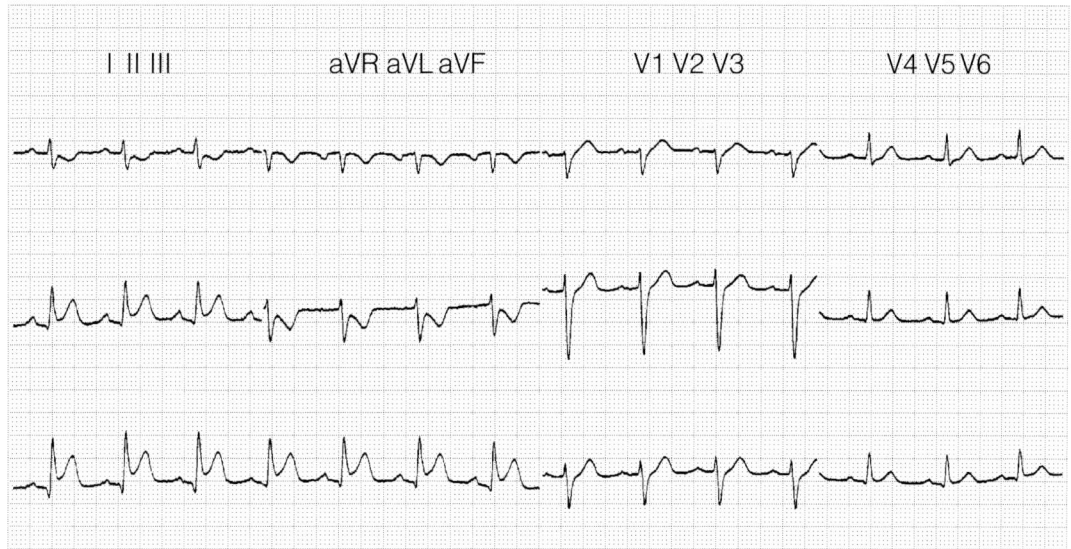

Figure 9.23. Practice tracing.

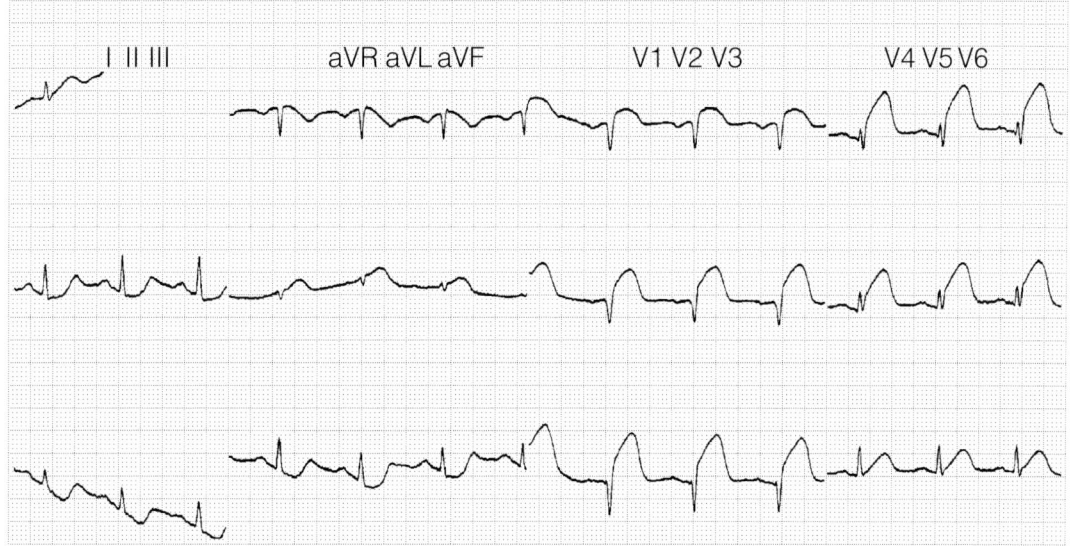

Figure 9.24. Practice tracing.

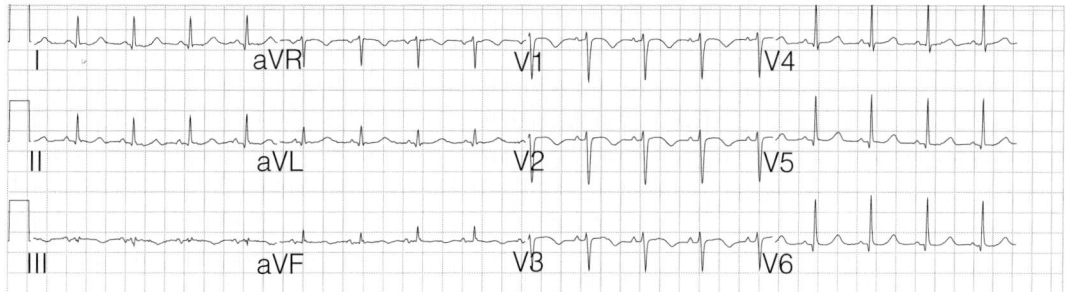

Figure 9.25. Practice tracing.

10

Ischemia and Anginal Syndromes

Not all instances of diminished coronary artery perfusion result in myocardial infarction. In Chapter 10, we will discuss ECG findings in less than complete coronary artery obstruction.

Pathophysiology of Ischemia

When arterial perfusion of tissue is inadequate to meet metabolic needs, we say that the tissue is *ischemic*. Metabolic needs, in the case of muscle, are dependent on the workload of that muscle.

In coronary artery disease, incomplete obstruction of the coronary arteries with atherosclerotic plaque limits myocardial perfusion. Under circumstances of rest, the diminished flow of oxygenated arterial blood may still be sufficient to meet the metabolic needs of the myocardium. However, during periods of exercise, the needs of the myocardium may require a greater volume of blood than can be delivered through the partially obstructed coronary arteries. In short, *myocardial oxygen consumption* may outstrip oxygen supply. The result is ischemia of the myocardium.

Anginal Syndromes

If the patient has chest pain in association with ischemia occurring during exercise, the syndrome is labeled *exertional angina pectoris*. Typically, when the patient rests, the imbalance between oxygen supply and demand resolves and the pain goes away.

Exercise is not the only circumstance under which angina can occur, however. Any circumstance that increases heart rate or blood pressure, for example, anxiety or a large meal, may increase myocardial oxygen consumption and result in angina.

Myocardial ischemia can also occur without producing chest pain. Many patients with coronary artery disease have frequent periods of *silent ischemia* occurring in the absence of chest pain.

Often in clinical practice we see patients who have prolonged periods of ischemic chest pain at rest, but who do not demonstrate evidence of AMI. This syndrome is called *unstable angina*. It typically occurs in patients with a very severe fixed *stenosis* or narrowing of a coronary artery, often exceeding a 90% obstruction. Sometimes a thrombus waxing and waning at the site of the stenosis will intermittently further narrow or occlude the lumen. A high percentage of these patients will go on to develop AMI.

Coronary artery spasm is another cause of myocardial ischemia, and has been labeled *variant angina* or *Prinzmetal's angina*. Variant angina can occur even in patients with completely clean coronary arteries, although, more often, spasm occurs in the immediate vicinity of atherosclerotic plaque in patients with coronary artery disease. Spasm diminishes perfusion and can produce exactly the same ischemic consequences as atherosclerosis.

Spasm, by definition, is intermittent and can cause transient chest pain. It seems to occur more often when the patient is at rest. Severe spasm that produces near total occlusion can produce ST-segment elevation that rises during spasm and subsides as the coronary artery spasm subsides.

Cocaine is a well-documented precipitator of coronary artery spasm that can induce a clinical picture of ischemic chest discomfort that is indistinguishable at presentation from other acute coronary syndromes. Typically, the patient presenting with cocaine-induced coronary spasm will be a male under 40 years of age, a smoker, will have used cocaine within several hours before the onset of symptoms, and will have few risk factors for coronary atherosclerosis. Approximately 6% of patients presenting with cocaine-induced coronary artery spasm will have spasm severe enough to produce necrosis and elevation of coronary biochemical markers.

Electrophysiologic Changes During Ischemia

During periods of ischemia, blood flow diminishes first and most dramatically in the subendocardium. Epicardial blood flow is preserved until the artery supplying the affected muscle becomes almost completely obstructed. As a result, ischemia usually involves only a partial thickness of the ventricular wall.

Significant metabolic changes occur in the ischemic inner wall (subendocardium), whereas the metabolic state of the outer wall (epicardium) remains nearly normal. This creates a difference in electrical potential between ischemic and normal tissue with the net result being that there is a current flow from normal cells in the epicardium toward the ischemic cells in the endocardium (Figure 10.1). This current flow takes place during mechanical systole, which, as you know from Chapter 1, occupies the time interval of the ST segment. Because the current is flowing away from ECG electrodes on the body surface overlying the affected ventricular wall, it is registered on the ECG as a negative needle deflection, resulting in *ST depression*. As you would surmise, these same electrophysiologic events can also alter T waves.

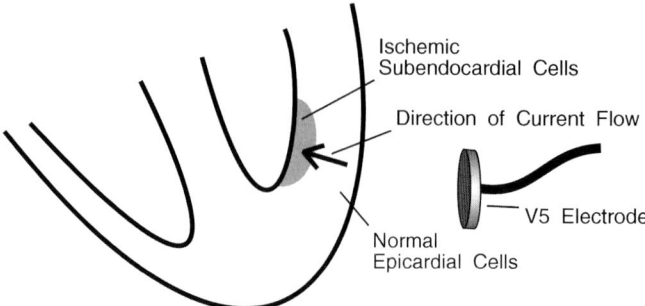

Figure 10.1. Schematic view of the left ventricle showing the flow of current during systole from healthy cells in the epicardium toward ischemic cells in the subendocardium. Note that the current flow is away from the V$_5$ electrode, producing a negative deflection of the ECG needle, which results in ST depression.

When ischemia involves the full thickness of the ventricular wall, that is, both endocardium and epicardium, we say that it is *transmural*. As noted above, this requires almost total cessation of blood flow through a coronary artery. *Transmural ischemia* produces ST elevation, with which you are already familiar from your study of AMI (Chapter 9).

Characteristics of Ischemic ST Depression

The ST-segment depression seen with nontransmural ischemia typically is either horizontal (flat) or downsloping, and the ST segment is usually quite straight, as shown in Figure 10.2. Also note that the ST segment in ischemia typically intersects with the T wave at a fairly abrupt angle. Both the straight ST segment and the abrupt transition into the T wave are in contrast to other causes of ST depression. Left ventricular hypertrophy, for example, has downsloping ST depression, but it is typically upwardly convex, and there is a gentle transition into the T wave (Figure 10.3).

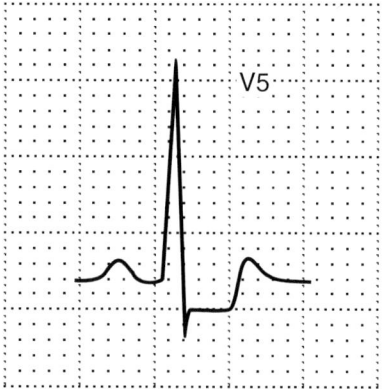

Figure 10.2. Ischemia. Horizontal ST-segment depression associated with ischemia. Note that the ST segment is quite straight and intersects with the T wave at a fairly sharp angle.

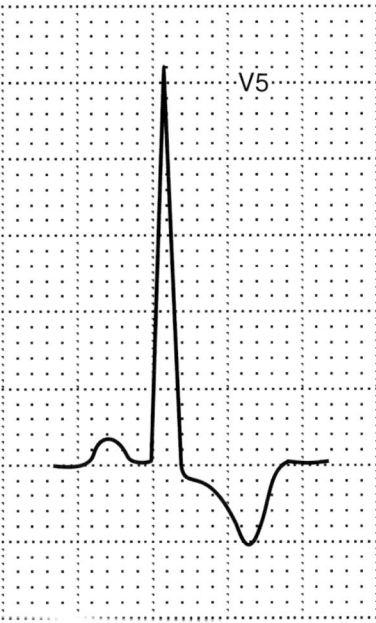

Figure 10.3. Left ventricular hypertrophy. Note that the ST depression in LVH is downsloping, as ischemia can be, but that the ST segment is convex as opposed to straight, and gently blends into the T wave.

Upsloping ST depression, on the other hand, much less often represents ischemia and, in fact, is quite normal during periods of exercise or other causes of tachycardia. This normal exertional ST depression is often referred to as *J point depression* (Figure 10.4).

ST depression is measured from the isoelectric line, usually established by the PR segment. As a general rule, the deeper the ST depression, the more

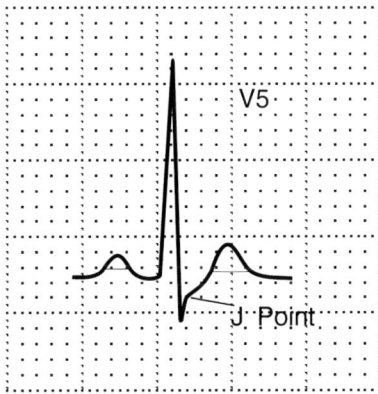

Figure 10.4. J point depression. Upsloping ST depression from the J point, which is a physiologic response to exercise or tachycardia.

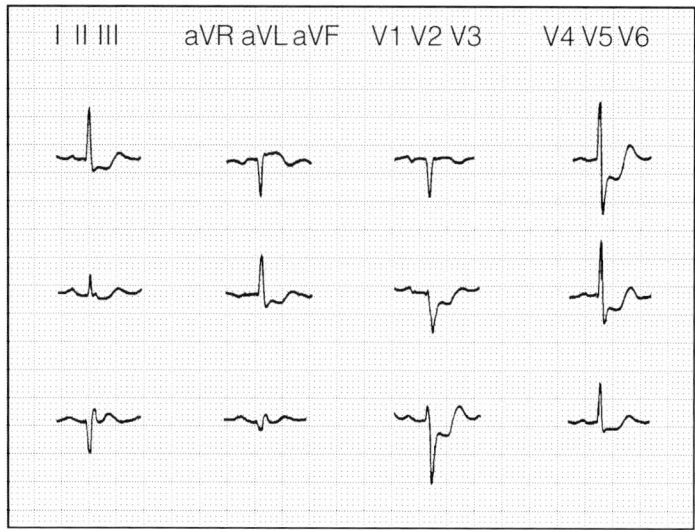

Figure 10.5. Ischemia. ECG of a 76-year-old white male recorded during an episode of angina. Note up to 3 mm of horizontal or downsloping ST depression in the anterolateral wall. In addition, pathologic Q waves are present in leads III and aVF, reflecting a previous inferior wall infarction.

severe the ischemia. In addition, the deeper the ST depression, the greater the specificity for ischemia. ST depression of <1 mm is an unreliable indicator of ischemia. Figure 10.5 shows the full 12-lead ECG of a patient with severe ischemia during an anginal attack.

Intermittent ST Depression

As you learned earlier in this chapter, ischemia is usually a changing, dynamic state that comes and goes, depending on the current balance or imbalance between oxygen supply and oxygen demand in the tissues. By the same token, ST depression is also often transient. It comes and goes with the ischemic state. Many patients with severe coronary artery disease display perfectly normal ECGs at rest and demonstrate ST depression only when ischemia is precipitated by exercise or occurs during an anginal episode. This fact gave rise to *exercise stress testing* as a means of detecting occlusive coronary artery disease in patients with normal resting ECGs. During stress testing, a 12-lead ECG is continuously monitored while the patient walks on a treadmill or peddles a stationary bicycle. Any ischemia provoked by exercise is then detected by observing for horizontal or downsloping ST depression of >1 mm. Care must be taken not to falsely interpret physiologic J point depression as representing ischemia.

Figure 10.6A shows the tracing of a 51-year-old white male with a normal resting ECG, diagnostic ST depression occurring at 10.5 min into exercise, and resolution of ST changes by 4 min into the postexercise period.

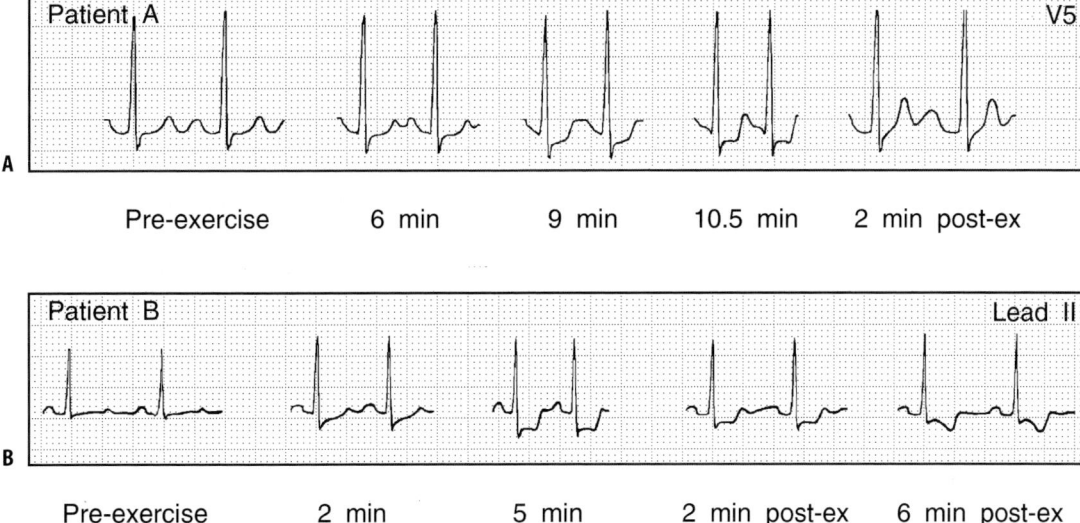

Figure 10.6. Exercise stress testing. **A.** Patient A is a 51-year-old white male with a history of atypical chest pain. Note that the ST segment is normal in the preexercise and postexercise tracings. However, by 10.5 min into exercise he shows approximately 2 mm of horizontal ST depression and an abrupt juncture with the T wave, which is typical of myocardial ischemia. **B.** Patient B is a 62-year-old white female with typical exertional chest discomfort who, in addition to horizontal ST depression, demonstrates T wave inversion by 6 min into the postexercise period. Note, however, that if the 6-minute postexercise tracing were viewed on an isolated ECG, it would be easy to confuse the ST and T wave changes with the strain pattern of LVH.

Chronic ST Depression

Some patients with coronary artery disease have persistent imbalances between oxygen supply and demand that are reflected as *chronic ST depression* on the ECG. Thus, these patients display ST depression even on the resting electrocardiogram in the absence of pain (Figure 10.7).

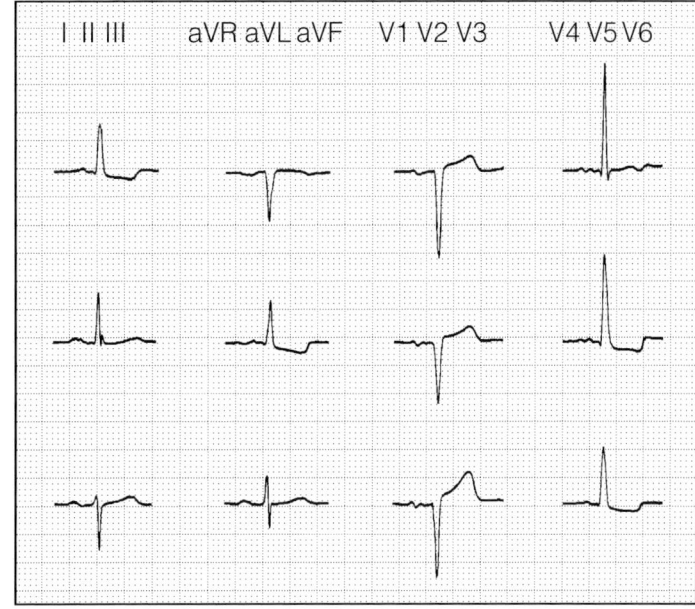

Figure 10.7. Chronic ST Depression. This 76-year-old male patient demonstrates chronic ST depression that persists from tracing to tracing in the high lateral wall (I, aVL, V_5, and V_6). Note that the downsloping ST depression forms an abrupt angle with the T wave, and that the T wave itself is altered by the ischemia. This patient also demonstrates evidence of a previous anterior myocardial infarction, in the form of pathologic Q waves in V_1–V_3.

T Wave Inversion

As briefly mentioned earlier in this chapter, the flow of current from normal myocardial cells in the epicardium toward ischemic cells in the subendocardium during systole can also change repolarization sequences, resulting in T wave abnormalities. Thus, *T wave inversion*, although seen less frequently than ST depression, is another potential indicator of ischemia. T wave inversion may accompany ST depression, or it may be seen alone as a manifestation of ischemia. Figure 10.6B shows T wave inversion occurring postexercise in a 62-year-old white female with typical exertional chest discomfort and a positive stress exercise test for ischemia. Note, however, that the upwardly convex nature of the ST depression gently sloping into an inverted T wave could easily be confused with LVH if viewed on an isolated ECG. Thus, T wave inversion is a less reliable indicator of ischemia than is horizontal ST depression.

Differential Diagnosis of ST Abnormalities

It should be clear by now that there are many conditions that can affect ST segments and T waves, including BBB, AMI, chamber enlargement, and ischemia. You will learn of even more in Chapter 13 (Miscellaneous Conditions). A frequent reader of ECGs will also see many tracings with mild ST abnormalities that can only be called *nonspecific ST and T wave changes* because they are not clearly characteristic of any of the conditions referred to above (Figure 10.8).

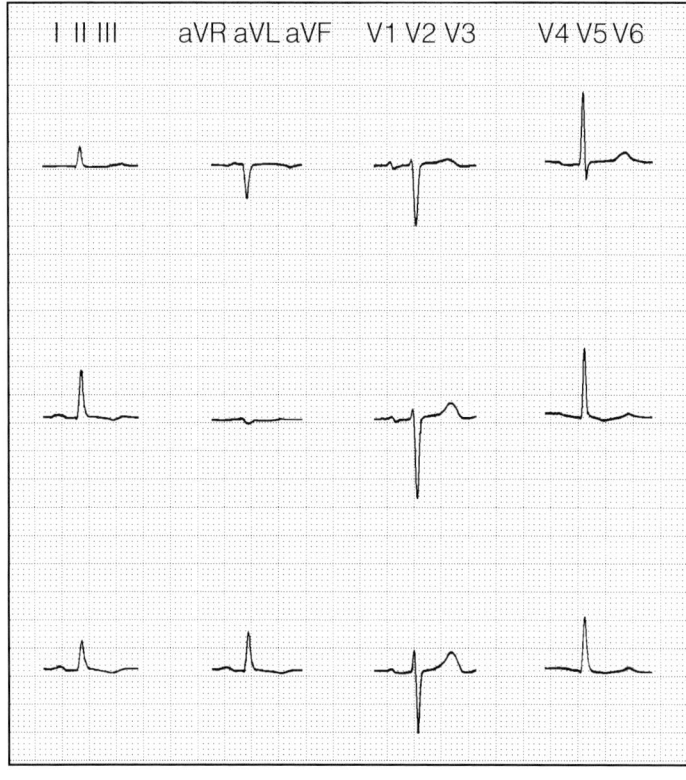

Figure 10.8. Nonspecific ST changes. Note that the sagging ST segments and minimal T wave inversion in the inferior and lateral walls are not clearly characteristic of any specific category of ST segment or T wave abnormality, thus, the designation "nonspecific."

A few hints can be helpful in sorting out these sometimes difficult differentiations. With regard to ischemia, perhaps the most helpful clue when evaluating ST and T wave abnormalities is whether or not they change from tracing to tracing. Conditions like BBB and LVH are persistent and do not change much over a period of time. Ischemic ST depression, however, frequently changes from tracing to tracing. Thus, as usual, it is a good idea to compare the current tracing to an old tracing on file whenever possible to see if noted changes are acute or chronic.

The straightness of the ST segment and the acuteness of the angle with the T wave are highly significant criteria when evaluating ST depression, and their presence makes the changes more likely to be ischemic in origin.

Finally, clinical correlation, as always, is also helpful. For example, ST depression appearing with chest pain and resolving when the chest pain resolves makes the diagnosis of ischemia a virtual certainty. The clinical and ECG correlates of ischemic heart disease will be the subject of our next chapter.

Practice Tracings

Several practice tracings (Figures 10.9 to 10.12) are included on this and the next page for honing your skills in diagnosing myocardial ischemia. The answers may be found in the Chapter 14.

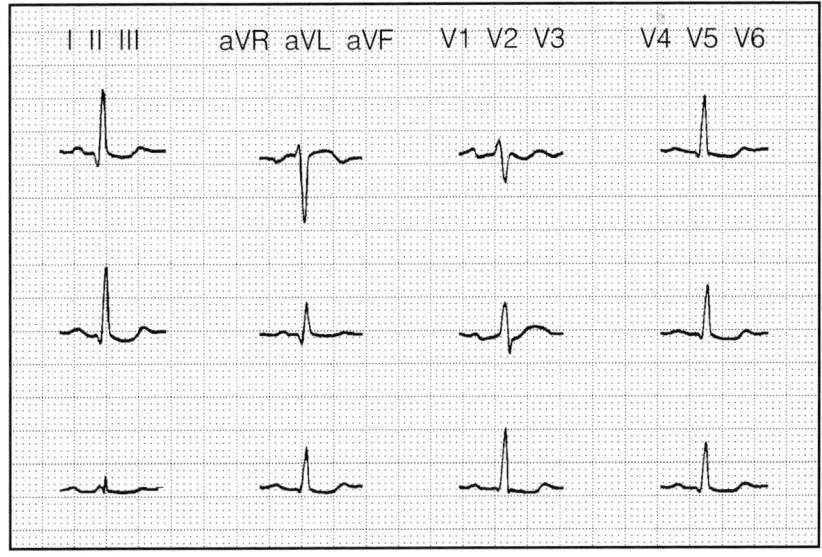

Figure 10.9. Practice tracing.

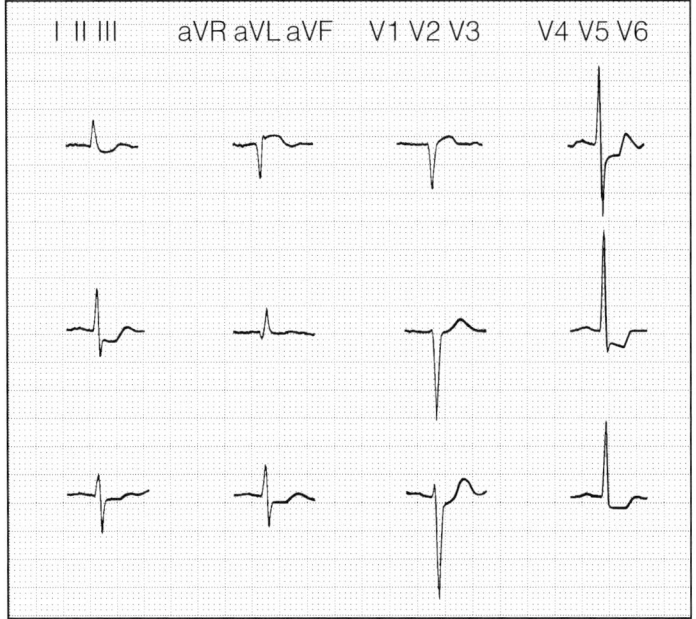

Figure 10.10. Practice tracing.

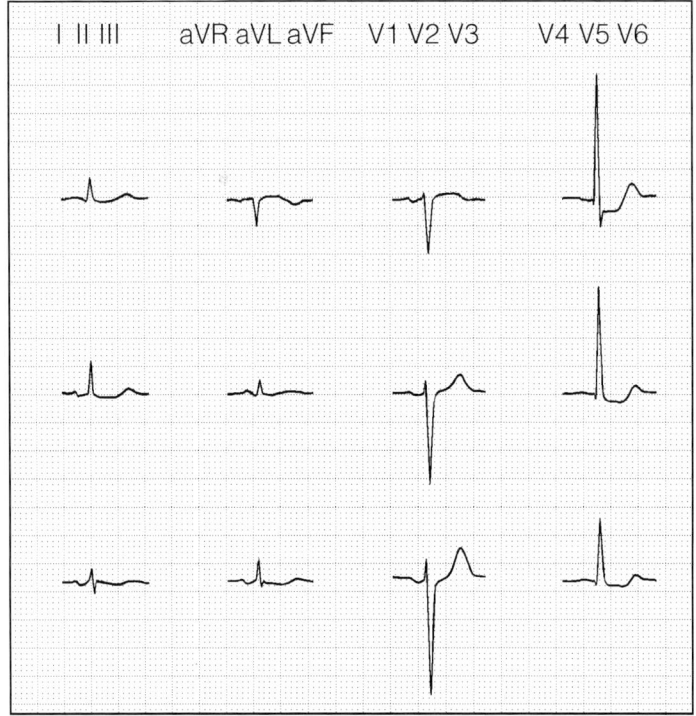

Figure 10.11. Practice tracing.

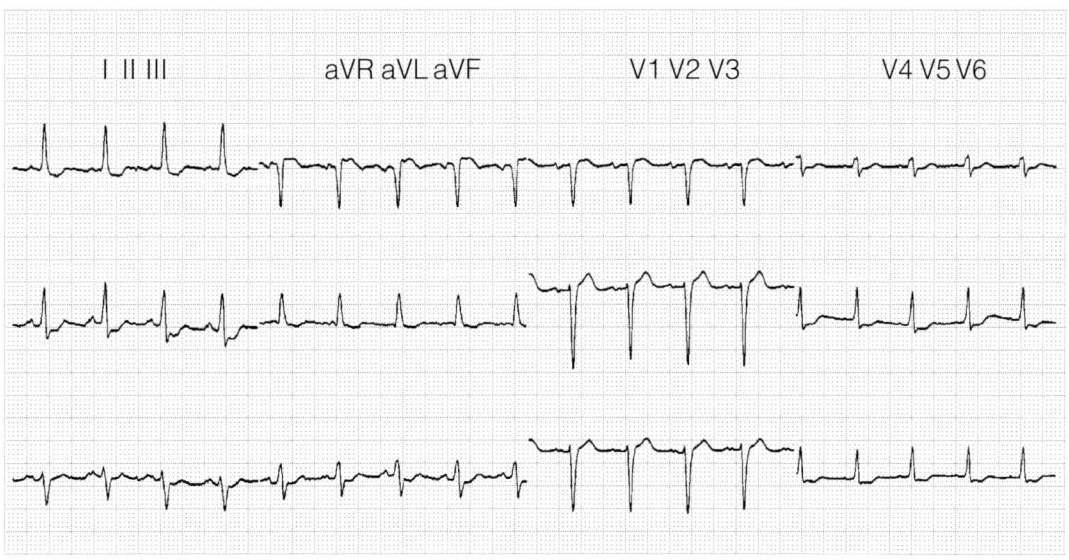

Figure 10.12. Practice tracing.

11

The Electrocardiogram and the Clinical Evaluation of Chest Pain

Interpretation of the 12-lead ECG is always more accurate when correlated with the patient's clinical presentation. In this chapter, we will discuss the various clinical syndromes of ischemic heart disease, the approach to the patient with chest pain, and the use of the ECG in chest pain evaluation.

The ECG as a Tool

Because there are often several diagnoses that can produce similar changes in the ECG, it is usually a mistake to rely on the ECG alone in making a diagnosis. Rather, it should be considered as just one of many pieces of evidence that must be weighed in reaching an accurate clinical diagnosis. Therefore, it is always important to interpret the ECG in light of the patient's clinical presentation.

For example, in Figure 9.17, you saw how patients with ventricular aneurysms frequently have persistent ST elevation that sometimes cannot easily be distinguished from that caused by an acute infarction. It would be very easy to mistakenly conclude that such a patient was having an acute infarction, unless we noted that the patient was pain free and had no symptoms compatible with AMI.

Correlation of the ECG with the clinical presentation is never more important than when approaching the patient with potential ischemic heart disease. In this chapter, we will discuss in detail the clinical presentation of the various syndromes associated with ischemic heart disease and the clinical approach to this group of patients.

The Role of History Taking

The clinical presentation of ischemic heart pain remains one of the most diverse in medicine. Nevertheless, studies have demonstrated that a history taken by an experienced clinician is a more accurate predictor of ischemic heart disease than any single available test, with the exception of coronary arteriography. For this reason, an accurate history taken by a well-trained ACLS provider is paramount to the evaluation of the patient presenting with chest pain. In most instances, it is the history that will trigger the provider's decision to move the patient along a path of evaluation for ischemic heart disease.

Syndromes of Ischemic Heart Disease

The continuum of ischemic heart disease stretches from silent ischemia through the various patterns of angina, AMI, and scars of a previous myocardial infarction, to the complications of AMI, such as ventricular aneurysm or pericarditis. Although all of these syndromes represent a continuum of the same disease process, they may present with quite different ECG patterns at different stages of the continuum, and have distinctly different treatments and outcomes. When a patient presents with chest pain, the ECG can help us to determine where they fit on the continuum. Similarly, the nature of the patient's symptoms and the physical examination can also provide clues as to where the patients fit on the continuum, and can lead us to search for subtle ECG changes that we might otherwise overlook without a high index of suspicion.

Stable Angina

Stable *exertional angina*, occurring predictably with a given level of exercise, is the most common initial presentation of ischemic heart disease. Discomfort appears with a fairly predictable and reproducible level of exercise, such as walking briskly for half a block, and just as predictably fades within several minutes with rest or nitroglycerin. The discomfort is variously described as a pressure, tightness, weight, band around the chest, indigestion, or gas. It may be felt in the epigastrium, retrosternally, in the arms, shoulders, neck, jaws, or even the back.

Occasionally, shortness of breath with exertion (in the absence of chronic lung disease) may be the only manifestation of angina. Nausea, vomiting, and diaphoresis are usually absent with angina.

Pathologically, stable angina is characterized by fixed obstructive coronary disease, usually requiring greater than a 50% stenosis. The prognosis for stable angina is quite good, and usually no emergency treatment other than sublingual nitroglycerin is required.

The ECG may or may not show evidence of ischemia, depending on the timing of the tracing. As you learned in Chapter 10, many patients with angina have perfectly normal tracings in the absence of pain. It is important to remember that a normal tracing in a patient whose pain has resolved does not rule out the diagnosis of angina. Every attempt should be made to perform the ECG while the patient has pain. It is, therefore, a matter of good practice to perform a 12-lead ECG before the administration of sublingual nitroglycerin in patients with chest pain.

Unstable Angina

Unstable angina is characterized by any change from a previous stable pattern of angina, or by new onset of angina. Frequent manifestations include discomfort coming with less and less exertion and discomfort coming at rest, lasting longer, or requiring more nitroglycerin for relief.

Duration of discomfort is frequently longer than with stable angina, and may last as long as an hour or more without the patient developing evidence of AMI. Nausea, vomiting, and diaphoresis are still typically absent, although, as with stable angina, shortness of breath may occasionally be present.

An interesting and not uncommon pattern is that of angina that occurs at rest after lying down, and is relieved by sitting up or by walking around the room. This *recumbent* or *nocturnal angina* is thought to be caused by an increase in cardiac work that occurs in the recumbent position because of increased venous return. Although recumbent angina usually represents a relatively severe degree of stenosis, there are patients for whom it represents a stable pattern, and it does not necessarily represent unstable angina.

Pathologically, unstable angina, (sometimes in older terminology called the *intermediate syndrome* when associated with prolonged pain), is typically characterized by severe fixed obstructive disease with stenosis often in excess of 90%. It is frequently precipitated by plaque rupture and the development of a nonocclusive thrombus; that is, a thrombus that produces <100% obstruction of the affected artery.

Patients with unstable angina are at much higher risk of progressing to myocardial infarction in the near term and should be hospitalized. As with all forms of angina, the ECG may not show ischemia once pain has resolved.

Coronary Artery Spasm and Transmural Ischemia

There is also a subgroup of patients who display coronary artery spasm, usually in the vicinity of an obstructive lesion, but sometimes even in patients with no occlusive coronary artery disease. Spasm may effectively produce a 100% occlusion of the affected coronary artery and can therefore cause transmural ischemia and ST elevation that is indistinguishable from that of AMI. For this reason it is important to give a therapeutic trial of nitroglycerin to patients with ECG evidence of transmural ischemia before concluding with certainty that a myocardial infarction is in progress. Patients with transmural ischemia on the basis of spasm will show resolution of ST elevation when nitroglycerin or a calcium channel blocker is administered. Those with complete obstruction from a thrombosis will not.

Acute Myocardial Infarction

The discomfort of AMI may be of the same character and location as both stable and unstable angina, but is frequently more intense; that is, the discomfort is perceived as hurting more. It may come with or without exertion and is unrelieved, or, at best, only partially relieved by rest or nitroglycerin.

Shortness of breath, nausea, vomiting, and diaphoresis are frequent, but not necessary, companions of AMI. Their presence, however, strengthens the presumption of AMI. Particularly powerful indicators of AMI are the presence of pain in the jaws or profound diaphoresis, and chest pain patients displaying such symptoms should be considered to have AMI until proven otherwise.

Other symptoms associated with acutely diminished cardiac output may also appear with AMI, including pallor, near syncope, and diminished men-

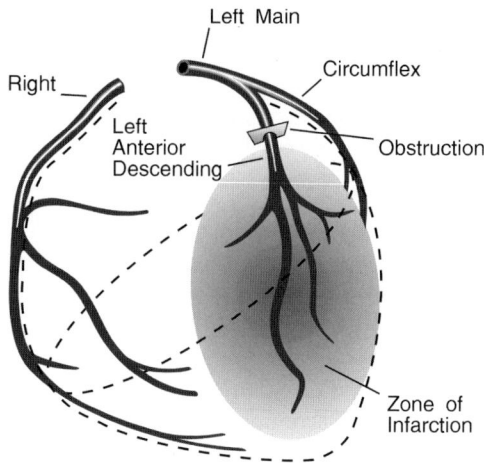

Figure 11.1. Proximal occlusion of the left anterior descending coronary artery producing a large zone of infarction.

tation. Of course, sudden death on the basis of ventricular fibrillation may also be the presenting symptom in up to 40% of patients, although AMI is not a necessary prerequisite of ventricular fibrillation.

Pathologically, AMI is the result of complete occlusion of the coronary lumen, most commonly by the development of a thrombus over a ruptured plaque in the diseased portion of the vessel. Muscle supplied by the affected vessel distal to the occlusion is in jeopardy of necrosis. Proximal occlusions affect a larger muscle mass than distal occlusions (Figures 11.1 and 11.2).

The quantity of muscle lost to necrosis in AMI is dependant upon the size of the affected vessel, the proximal or distal location of the lesion, and the quantity of collateral circulation from other vessels to the muscle in jeopardy. Loss of >40% of ventricular muscle in AMI generally results in cardiogenic shock and death.

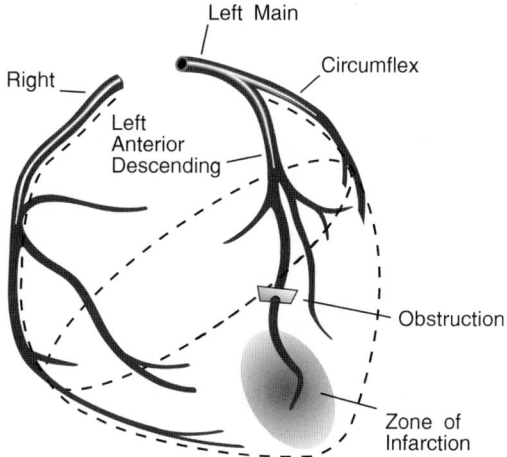

Figure 11.2. Distal occlusion of the left anterior descending producing a much smaller zone of infarction than is seen with proximal occlusions

You are by now well familiar with the ECG changes of AMI. Remember, however, that occasionally in the early stages of either transmural (STEMI) or nontransmural (NSTEMI) AMI the ECG may remain negative and not show evidence of infarction for hours. Occasionally, patients with AMI may complete their infarction and never show clear ECG evolution of AMI. This is another reason why a high index of suspicion on the basis of the patient's history is so important.

Acute Coronary Syndrome

The term acute coronary syndrome refers to a category of patients presenting with chest discomfort in whom there is a high clinical index of suspicion that the source of the chest discomfort is ischemic heart disease. This category encompasses patients with unstable angina, NSTEMI, and STEMI. It is a useful term clinically because often the source of chest discomfort is not clear at the time of presentation, and deciding that the patient has to be approached as potentially being an acute coronary syndrome determines the pathway of evaluation and treatment that we will follow. More on that in a later chapter.

Taking the History

It is apparent from the present discussion that the following are essential baseline questions that must be asked of any patient with chest pain:

1. When did the discomfort begin?
2. Where do you feel it?
3. Does it travel anyplace?
4. How would you describe the discomfort?
5. Has the discomfort been constant, or does it come and go?
6. Does it feel like any discomfort you have had in the past?
7. Is there anything that seems to aggravate the discomfort, or relieve the discomfort?
8. Did you break out in a sweat, have nausea or vomiting, or become short of breath?

This list is not exhaustive, of course, but answers to these questions should be considered the minimum quantity of information necessary to elicit an adequate history of chest pain. The questions can be asked while other tasks are being performed, and should not be permitted to delay essential care or transport.

Historical factors mitigating against a diagnosis of ischemic heart pain include:

- discomfort that repeatedly comes at rest, but not with exercise
- discomfort that goes away with exercise
- discomfort on only one side of the chest, but not retrosternally
- pain that is described as "sharp like a knife"
- pain that lasts only seconds at a time

- pain that "flies in" and "flies out"
- pain that lasts for hours or days at a time in the obvious absence of myocardial infarction
- pain that is pleuritic (increases with respiration)

None of these historical factors, however, should be considered to safely rule out AMI. All of us with experience in diagnosing AMI have been misled by a history that seemed incompatible with AMI. The important factor in avoiding a missed diagnosis of AMI is to maintain a high index of suspicion.

Role of the Physical Examination

The role of the physical examination in the diagnosis of AMI should be viewed primarily as helping to lend confirmation to a diagnosis made primarily on the basis of history. It is not uncommon for the patient presenting with AMI to have an essentially normal preliminary cardiovascular examination. Therefore, it is important not to dismiss the diagnosis of AMI, or to lower the index of suspicion for AMI, simply on the basis of a normal physical examination.

Findings supporting a diagnosis of AMI include pallor, cold and clammy skin, diaphoresis, and an S_4 gallop. Patients who have developed *forward failure* (low cardiac output) as a complication of AMI may also display diminished pulses, hypotension, decreased mentation, and anxiety. Signs of *backward failure* (pulmonary edema) include prominent dyspnea, jugular venous distension, use of the accessory muscles of inspiration, rales, and an S_3 gallop.

Dysrhythmias common to AMI may be discovered at the time of auscultation or may be viewed on a cardiac monitor, and include ventricular ectopy, sinus bradycardia or tachycardia, atrial fibrillation, and the full spectrum of AV blocks.

Clinical Patterns of STEMI

Two major clinical categories of STEMI exist, each with their own characteristic clinical pattern based on the geographic distribution of the infarction, and the cardiac structures involved.

You will recall that the left coronary artery supplies the anterior wall of the left ventricle and is the principle source of blood supply to the septum and, therefore, the Bundle of His and the bundle branches.

The *right coronary artery* supplies the inferior or diaphragmatic portion of the left ventricle and, in most patients, supplies the SA and the AV nodes. It also supplies the right ventricle.

Anterior Wall STEMI

Anterior myocardial infarction occurs as the result of occlusion in the distribution of the left coronary artery. It is commonly a larger infarction, and may be associated with sinus tachycardia, pump failure, higher degrees of heart block (Mobitz type II or third degree), or with new BBB.

Higher degrees of heart block occurring with anterior myocardial infarction carry a bad prognosis because they are usually the result of extensive infarction with necrosis of the ventricular septum and the bundle of His or the bundle branches. Pacing is usually required for these higher degrees of heart block, but rarely alters outcome because these patients typically die of pump failure as a consequence of the extensive nature of the infarction.

Inferior Wall STEMI

Inferior myocardial infarction occurs with occlusion of the right coronary artery. It is commonly associated with a significant *vasovagal response* characterized by marked sinus bradycardia and hypotension that is usually responsive to atropine and volume expansion. Sinus bradycardia may be further aggravated by a diminution in perfusion to the SA node.

AV block, when seen with inferior myocardial infarction, is typically lower grade (first degree or Mobitz type I) and is the result of *edema* of the AV node, as opposed to necrosis. Because the level of block is in the AV node, even when block advances to third degree there is typically a reliable junctional escape rhythm present. Pacing is not usually required, and symptomatic bradycardia can usually be adequately treated with atropine. Pump failure is less often a problem than with anterior myocardial infarction, unless the patient has a more extensive than usual right coronary circulation or has lost muscle mass from a previous myocardial infarction.

Patients presenting with evidence of inferior myocardial infarction and isolated right heart failure (jugular venous distention and hypotension with clear lungs), should also have an ECG with V_3 and V_4 placed in their corresponding positions on the right side of the chest to rule out a right ventricular infarction.

Role of Serial ECGs and Continuous ST-Segment Monitoring

Earlier in this chapter, we discussed how the ECG may be negative in the early stages of NSTEMI or STEMI. It is often prudent in patients who have negative ECGs, but a high index of suspicion for acute coronary syndrome, to perform serial ECGs over a period of time.

Many emergency departments and coronary care units have monitoring equipment capable of continuous ST segment monitoring and trend analysis. This represents the ideal tool for evaluation of this category of patient because the emergency department staff become immediately aware of any ST-segment change. In the absence of continuous ST-segment monitoring, however, leaving the patient connected to the ECG machine and performing serial tracings every 10 to 15 min during the acute period is almost as useful.

Many hospitals have established chest pain evaluation centers, which incorporate approximately 9 hours of observation, serial ECGs (or continuous ST-segment monitoring), and serial cardiac enzyme determinations into their evaluation of patients with chest pain of unclear etiology.

12

The Advanced Cardiac Life Support Provider and Therapeutic Interventions in Acute Myocardial Infarction

It is important for an ACLS provider to become adept at rapidly identifying and preparing candidates for rapid intervention aimed at clearing the obstructed coronary artery with either pharmacologic thrombolysis or percutaneous coronary intervention (PCI) (balloon angioplasty and stenting). The ACLS provider can play a major role in improving the time between patient presentation and administration of these interventions.

Pathogenesis of AMI

In the mid 1960s, most respected pathologists held the view that AMI was the result of fixed obstructive disease of the coronary arteries, and that clot formation rarely played a role in AMI. In fact, at that time the old term *coronary thrombosis* was dropped from the lexicon, and the familiar term *myocardial infarction* substituted in its place.

Studies performed in the 1970s and 1980s, however, confirmed that an *acute thrombosis* occurring at the site of a ruptured atherosclerotic plaque was, indeed, the source of obstruction in over 85% of patients suffering AMI.[1] These studies rekindled interest in the concept of thrombolysis, ultimately resulting in a revolution in the approach to AMI.

The time required for complete necrosis of involved muscle to occur after complete coronary artery occlusion is variable, and it is dependent on the presence or absence of significant *collateral circulation* and a blood pressure adequate to perfuse those collaterals. Necrosis proceeds from endocardium to epicardium (Figure 12.1). Completion of necrosis, dependent on the aforementioned variables, may take from 1 to more than 6 hours (Figures 12.1 and 12.2). Younger people have fewer years over which to develop collateral circulation to ischemic areas and may necrose muscle faster than older patients. Unfortunately, an AMI in a 40-year-old may constitute the worst case of the three necrosis curves, as shown in Figure 12.2, and young patients without collaterals may lose over 1% of salvageable myocardium per minute.

Although the usual case of straightforward STEMI falls within these time parameters of necrosis, there is a subgroup of patients who have what is often

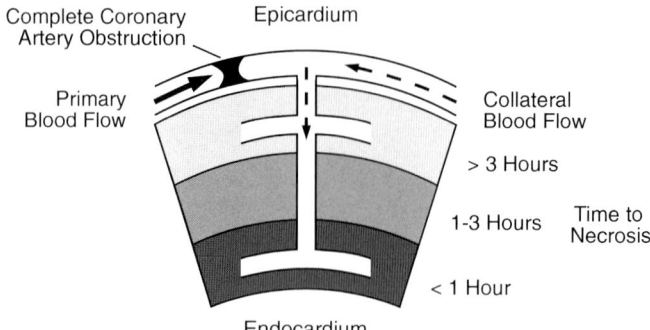

Figure 12.1. Schematic diagram showing the order of necrosis through the ventricular wall in AMI. Note that the endocardium necroses much faster than the epicardium because of less abundant collateral circulation. (Modified from Swan HJC, Anderson JL, et al. Practical Aspects of Thrombolysis in the Clinical Management of Acute Myocardial Infarction. American College of Cardiology.)

called a *stuttering pattern* of infarction. These patients demonstrate a stuttering or intermittent pattern of pain over as long as 24 hours or more, and their muscle seems to necrose more slowly than usual. Such a pattern probably reflects the waxing and waning of a thrombus undergoing natural thrombolysis, and then repropagation under the influence of the body's plasmin and plasminogen system.

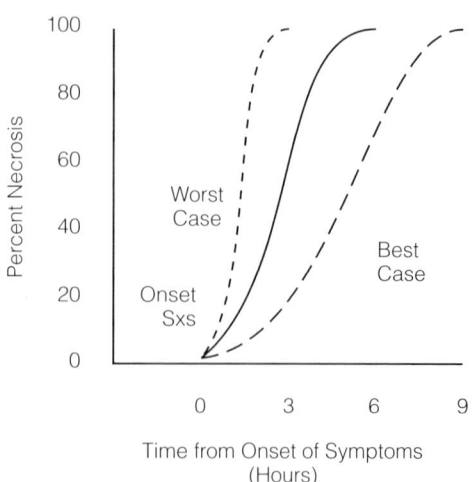

Figure 12.2. Graph depicting the percentage of necrosis in AMI as a function of time in the worst case, average case, and best case scenarios. Unfortunately, younger people often constitute the worst case because they have had less time to develop collateral circulation than older patients. (Modified from Swan HJC, Anderson JL, et al: Practical Aspects of Thrombolysis in the Clinical Management of Acute Myocardial Infarction. American College of Cardiology.)

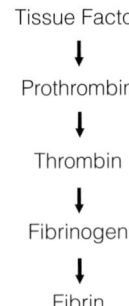

Coagulation Cascade

Tissue Factor

Prothrombin

Thrombin

Fibrinogen

Fibrin

Figure 12.3. The coagulation cascade.

Thrombus Formation

There are two major steps in thrombus formation. The first is called *primary hemostasis* and involves the activation of platelets in response to substances released by the exposed interior of a ruptured plaque. These substances include lipids, collagen, and tissue factor. The platelets adhere to collagen fibers in the vascular endothelium and form a platelet "plug." Platelets are then linked together by fibrinogen. *Glycoprotein IIb/IIIa* is an essential component of these links. Drugs called *IIb/IIIa inhibitors* block these links and help inhibit growth of the platelet aggregate.

The second major step is called *secondary hemostasis*, in which the complex *coagulation cascade* is initiated. The ultimate goal of the cascade is to produce cross-linked fibrin, which is the heart of a clot. In brief, the major elements of the cascade are the release of tissue factor, which ultimately activates prothrombin, which is then converted to thrombin. Thrombin, in turn, converts fibrinogen to fibrin. The basics of this cascade are illustrated in Figure 12.3.

Reperfusion Strategies

The ultimate goal of therapeutic interventions in STEMI is to rapidly reestablish perfusion of the myocardium affected by an AMI, thereby salvaging myocardium that would otherwise necrose and die. Two major categories of *reperfusion* therapy exist. The first is pharmacologic reperfusion, utilizing a variety of drugs that lyse a thrombus, and the second is the physical opening of an occluded coronary artery with balloon angioplasty or stenting. The latter is often called *PCI.*

Which strategy should be chosen? As the old saying goes, timing is everything. We have already learned that "time is muscle," and that the longer a coronary occlusion persists, the more muscle is lost. In general, when the time from patient presentation to either "needle" (for thrombolysis) or "balloon" (for PCI) is <90 min, PCI is the preferable strategy, resulting in slightly lower absolute mortality. Furthermore, the sicker the patient (i.e., the higher on the Killip class scale), the greater the benefit of PCI, to the extent

Table 12.1. Killup Classification of Heart Failure

Class I	No clinical heart failure
Class II	Rales $\frac{1}{2}$ way up lung fields
Class III	Rales in all lung fields (pulmonary edema)
Class IV	Cardiogenic shock; BP > 90 systolic; pulmonary edema

that for Killip (Table 12.1) class 4 patients in cardiogenic shock the evidence favoring PCI is compelling, as shown in the SHOCK trial.[2,3]

Because thrombi become more resistant to fibrinolytic therapy with the passage of time, the efficacy of thrombolysis is greatest in patients receiving treatment within the first 2–3 hours after onset of symptoms. PCI is less time dependent because restoring arterial patency is more reliable with PCI than with thrombolysis, especially in older thrombi in patients who have had symptoms for longer than 3 hours. Thus, in patients who have had symptoms for longer than 3 hours, primary PCI becomes more clearly the preferable choice, if it can be accomplished within 90 min.

PCI may also be favored in those patients at higher risk for bleeding with thrombolytics, or those with other contraindications to thrombolysis. Patients over the age of 75 are three times more likely to experience death, reinfarction, or stroke after fibrinolysis than with PCI.

Nevertheless, when door-to-balloon time would exceed 90 min, or when the difference between needle time and balloon time would exceed 60 min (even when under the 90 minute limit for PCI), evidence suggests that thrombolysis may still be the preferable intervention.

Obviously, which strategy will result in the quickest and most reliable end result of reperfusion is the key. Thus, many factors impose on the decision of which category of reperfusion to select, primary among which are the duration of symptoms and the availability of facilities for performing rapid PCI. For those hospitals offering immediate 24-hour availability of emergency PCI, the answer is easy. For others without cardiac catheterization laboratories, the decision involves calculations of transport time to a facility capable of emergent PCI versus the benefits of immediate pharmacologic thrombolysis. Each hospital emergency department needs to give careful consideration to all factors and develop written protocols that speed patient management decisions.

Pharmacologic Reperfusion: The Value of Thrombolytic Agents in STEMI

The goal of thrombolytic therapy is the reperfusion of coronary arteries acutely occluded by a thrombus. Studies have shown that reperfusion with thrombolytics can result in striking reductions in mortality, in the range of 20% to 52%, with the greatest benefit seen in those patients receiving thrombolytic therapy within 70 min of the onset of symptoms.[4-7] In the early GISSI studies, mortality was reduced by 47% if therapy was initiated within 1 hour of onset of symptoms, by 23% if within 3 hours, and by 17% if between 3 and 6 hours (Figure 12.4).[8] More recently, other studies have suggested benefit even after 6 hours in some patients, and the American College of Cardiology

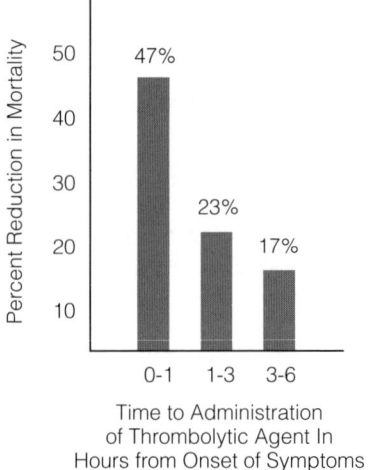

Figure 12.4. Percentage of reduction in mortality from AMI reported in the GISSI study as a function of the time to administration of a thrombolytic agent from onset of symptoms. Note that benefit of therapy drops off sharply after the first hour.

(ACC)/American Heart Association (AHA) guidelines currently support treatment within 12 hours from onset of symptoms of STEMI, and up to 24 hours for patients with evidence of ongoing ischemia, such as a stuttering pattern of pain.[9–12]

Studies have also demonstrated improvement in *left ventricular function* following thrombolytic therapy, but these benefits are less striking than the improvement in mortality.[10]

The Early Treatment of AMI

The advent of thrombolytic therapy increased the importance of rapid and accurate evaluation of chest pain, including, of course, evaluation of an ECG. Unfortunately, as previously noted, the benefits of therapy are exquisitely time dependent.

Many patients still do not achieve maximum benefit because of delays in administration of therapy. Although patient delays in seeking care account for the single largest component of delay (averaging approximately two hours), events after the patient has entered the medical care system constitute the causes of delay of greatest magnitude that are potentially rapidly correctable.

The development of chest pain protocols that include an early ECG, particularly a prehospital ECG, have significantly reduced in-hospital delays. ACC Guidelines set a goal of administering thrombolytic therapy within 30 min of patient arrival, a period sometimes referred to as the *golden half hour*. One of the important skills of an ACLS provider is to become adept at rapidly identifying candidates for reperfusion therapy and preparing them for intervention.

Thrombolytic Agents

Thrombolytic agents (also called *fibrinolytics*) are *plasminogen activators* which convert naturally occurring plasminogen to plasmin, and are able to actively dissolve, or *lyse*, thrombi, as opposed to simply preventing thrombus propagation, as does heparin. Streptokinase, alteplase (t-PA), reteplase, and tenecteplase have enjoyed the widest use. Streptokinase, despite producing a systemic lytic state as compared to the other more fibrin-specific drugs, has a slightly lower incidence of intracranial hemorrhage, but also has a lower 90-minute patency rate and produces lower TIMI flow rates through reperfused coronary arteries.

The incidence of intracranial hemorrhage is <1% with all agents. Slightly more than 25% of patients will have mild-to-moderate systemic bleeding complications.[10,14,15] Streptokinase can produce allergic reactions (3.6%) or hypotensive reactions (up to 10%), but they are rarely severe.[10] Antibodies to streptokinase limit its effectiveness on a second occasion, and a previous exposure to streptokinase is an indication for the utilization of one of the other agents.

More important than which thrombolytic is used is how quickly it is administered.

Adjunctive Therapy

Remarkably, an aspirin, chewed immediately, augmented the reduction in mortality seen with streptokinase in the ISIS-2 study by an additional 20%.[9] In addition, aspirin reduced the incidence of nonfatal reinfarction and nonfatal stroke. The primary role of aspirin is to inhibit platelet aggregation, the event initiating thrombus formation in AMI. Because of its safety and remarkable efficacy, large public education campaigns have encouraged patients to chew an aspirin when encountering symptoms of chest pain potentially compatible with AMI.

Because the lysing of a fibrin clot with thrombolytics releases many potent activators of both platelets and the coagulation cascade, paradoxically, the administration of fibrinolytic drugs actually sets the stage for further thrombus formation. For this reason, unfractionated heparin or low molecular weight heparin are utilized by most clinicians during thrombolysis to inhibit the coagulation cascade. Heparin administered simultaneously with thrombolytic drugs has improved reperfusion rates.[15]

These antithrombin drugs are used in an effort to prevent reocclusion and to help protect the distal myocardial microvasculature from thrombin and platelet microemboli during clot lysis. Glycoprotein IIb/IIIa platelet aggregation inhibitors have also been used for the same reasons, sometimes in combination with half-dose thrombolytics, and routinely in patients undergoing angioplasty and stent placement. *Combination pharmacologic therapy* with a fibrinolytic and a IIb/IIIa inhibitor followed by immediate PCI is being studied, and may in the future become a favored intervention in patients who present within 3 hours.

There is no contraindication to using other traditional therapies during thrombolytic therapy, including nitroglycerin, beta blockers, calcium channel antagonists, and antiarrhythmics.

Reperfusion

Reperfusion after thrombolytic therapy may be manifested by prompt relief of pain, decrease in ST-segment elevation, reperfusion arrhythmias, early "washout" of enzymes, and, occasionally, signs of improved left ventricular function. Reperfusion dysrhythmias, which may include both atrial and ventricular ectopy, are usually short lived and rarely require treatment. An accelerated idioventricular rhythm is particularly common. Nevertheless, continuous monitoring during thrombolytic therapy is imperative.

The time it takes to reperfuse is highly variable, ranging from 5 min to 2–3 hours, but most patients reperfuse within the first hour. The incidence of reperfusion as a result of intravenous thrombolytic therapy is generally accepted to be over 70%, and in some studies it has exceeded 90%.

Reperfusion is usually accompanied by diminution of ST-segment elevation, particularly in cases that reperfuse early. Figure 12.5A is the tracing of a 59-year-old white male with acute inferior wall myocardial infarction taken at 9:23 AM during administration of streptokinase. Figure 12.5B is from the same patient, taken 7 min later at 9:30 AM, after sudden relief of pain. Note that substantial resolution of both ST-segment elevation and reciprocal depression has occurred with reperfusion. Late reperfusion, after substantial necrosis has occurred, is less likely to produce resolution of ECG changes.

Complications of Therapy

The most significant adverse reaction to thrombolytic therapy is, of course, bleeding. *Intracranial bleeding* is the most serious complication (<1%), but in actuality represents approximately the same incidence of stroke as occurs in control groups with AMI.[16] The overall incidence of bleeding is <5% when patients with uncontrolled hypertension and cerebrovascular disease are excluded. Nevertheless, special measures are warranted in the care of patients undergoing thrombolysis to reduce exogenous stimuli to bleeding, such as needlepricks and invasive procedures.

Dosing on the basis of body weight has reduced the incidence of bleeding with certain fibrinolytics.

Contraindications

As the relative safety and efficacy of thrombolytic therapy has become more clearly established, the number of absolute and relative contraindications has diminished. Age, for example, is no longer an obstacle to therapy. In the ISIS-2 study, patients as old as 90 years were treated, and there was a 32% mortality reduction with thrombolysis among patients in the over-70 age group.[9] Nevertheless, as mentioned earlier, composite indices of death, reinfarction, and cerebral bleeding are higher in older patients with fibrinolysis than with PCI, and PCI may be favored in the elderly when available within the 90-minute time window.

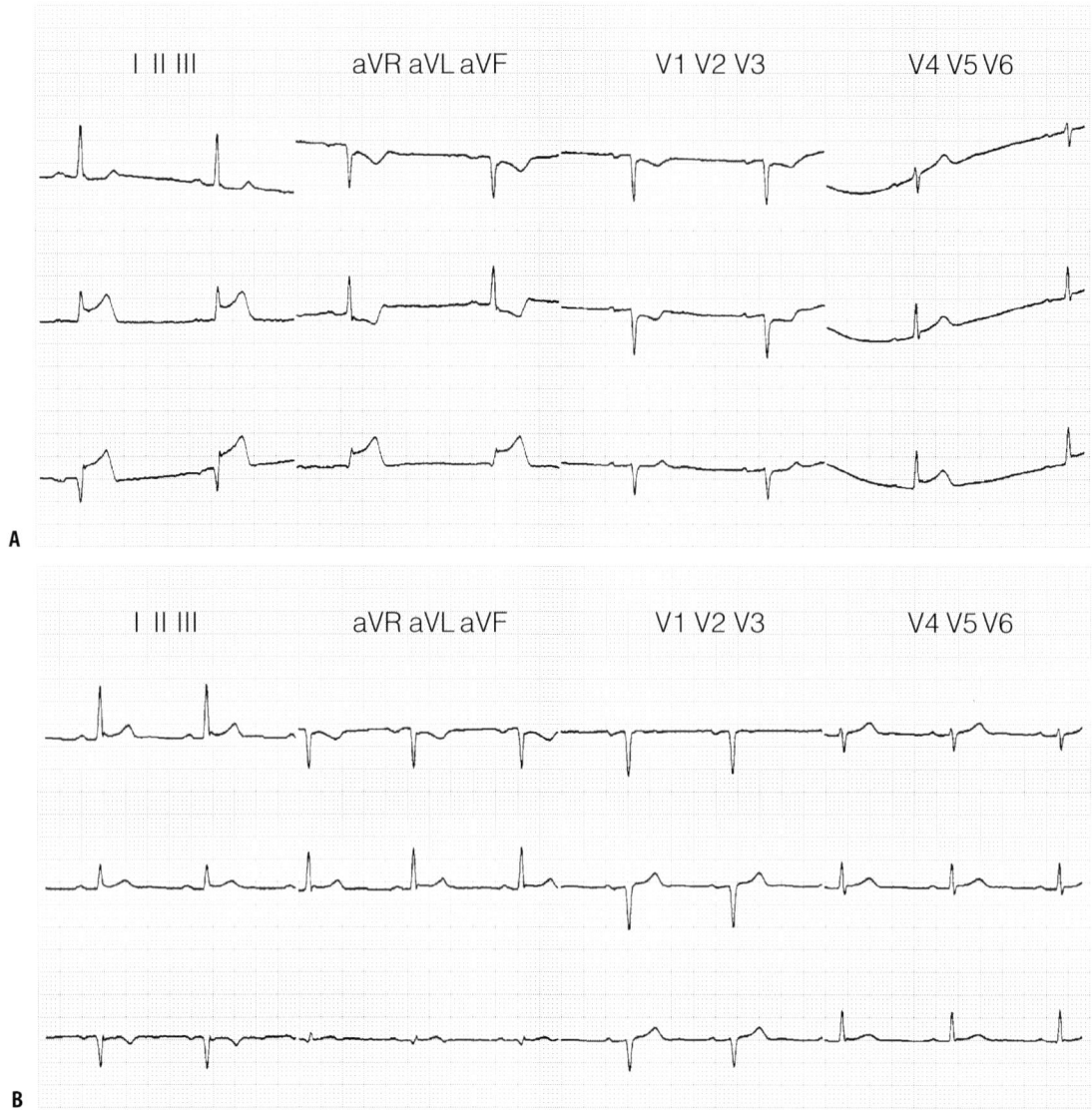

Figure 12.5 A. Tracing from a 59-year-old white male taken at 9:23 AM during streptokinase administration for acute inferior wall myocardial infarction. Note typical prominent ST elevation in the inferior wall, with reciprocal depression in leads I, aVL, and V_1 and V_2. **B.** Second tracing from the same patient taken 7 min later, at 9:30 AM, after sudden relief of pain. Note substantial resolution of ST-segment elevation and reciprocal depression that has occurred with reperfusion.

Absolute Contraindications

- Any prior intracranial hemorrhage
- Known structural cerebral vascular lesion (e.g., AV malformation)
- Malignant intracranial neoplasm
- Ischemic stroke in last 3 months
- Suspected aortic dissection
- Active bleeding or bleeding diathesis
- Closed head or facial trauma in last 3 months

Relative Contraindications

- Recent (3 weeks) major surgery
- Recent (3 weeks) trauma
- Cardiopulmonary resuscitation of >10 min
- BP > 180/110
- Ischemic stroke more than 3 months old
- Internal bleeding in last month
- Noncompressible vascular punctures
- For streptokinase/Anistreplase: prior exposure or allergy
- Pregnancy
- Active peptic ulcer
- Currently on anticoagulants (sodium warfarin, Coumadin); the higher the INR, the higher the risk

Some authors also exclude patients in pulmonary edema and cardiogenic shock (Killip Class III and IV) from consideration for thrombolysis because of the absence of statistically significant benefit from thrombolysis in this group of patients. Mortality rates in cardiogenic shock are more positively impacted by emergency PCI, which should constitute the treatment of choice whenever possible.[15] Nevertheless, the presence of pulmonary edema or cardiogenic shock should not be considered an absolute contraindication.

Identifying Candidates for Thrombolysis

Potential Candidates for Thrombolytic Therapy Include:

1. Persons of any age
2. History compatible with AMI
3. Duration of pain <12 hours
4. ECG compatible with AMI
5. No absolute contraindications.

It is not necessary or even desirable to confirm STEMI with enzyme (biochemical marker) determinations. Indeed, reliance on laboratory testing for confirmation of diagnosis is one of the causes of unnecessary delays in administration of therapy.

ECG criteria for compatibility with STEMI should include ST elevation of 1 mm or greater in at least two contiguous (adjacent) limb leads or elevation of 2 mm or greater in at least two contiguous precordial leads.

You learned in Chapter 9 that the changes of LBBB can simulate, but can also mask, an acute anterior myocardial infarction. For this reason, patients presenting with new LBBB and a history compatible with AMI should also be strongly considered for thrombolytic therapy.

As we learned in Chapter 10, patients with true posterior myocardial infarction may also be having a transmural STEMI, in which the evolutionary changes of AMI are actually manifested in the mirror image changes of tall R waves and ST-segment depression in the anterior leads of V_1–V_3. Although the data are insufficient to draw clear conclusions, the ACC/AHA guidelines assert that it may be reasonable to consider patients with such ECG findings as a STEMI equivalent, and, therefore, as potential candidates for reperfusion strategies.[12]

Finally, you have also learned that ST elevation is evanescent, that is, it comes and goes. Patients may present with Q waves and T wave inversion after the ST elevation has resolved and still be within the required time frames for administration of thrombolytic agents.

In summary, patients with the following ECG criteria should be considered for thrombolytic therapy:

1. ST elevation 1 mm or greater in 2 contiguous limb leads
2. ST elevation 2 mm or greater in 2 contiguous precordial leads
3. LBBB, particularly if new
4. New pathologic Q waves and T wave inversion in patients who clinically are still within the time windows for thrombolysis.

Remember that to avoid a mistaken diagnosis of AMI with each of these ECG criteria, it is important to have a history compatible with AMI. It is particularly important to screen for historical factors that might be compatible with an aortic dissection because administration of thrombolytic agents to these patients will likely constitute a fatal error. These factors include pain that is described as ripping, tearing, or searing, often with radiation to the back or lower extremities. The pain of aortic dissection is typically worst at onset and lasts for hours, but may gradually improve over those hours.

Potential clues of aortic dissection on physical examination include absence of any individual major pulses in the carotids or extremities, or a diastolic murmur of aortic regurgitation.

In addition, to avoid administering thrombolytics to patients who have transmural ischemia and ST-segment elevation on the basis of coronary artery spasm alone, it is important to administer a brief therapeutic trial of nitroglycerin before concluding that the patient has an AMI.

Percutaneous Coronary Intervention

Percutaneous coronary intervention (PCI) encompasses all of those procedures that can be accomplished via catheters inserted percutaneously. Balloon angioplasty and stent placement are the primary modalities utilized to physically open an occluded or partially obstructed coronary artery.

Improvements in mortality and morbidity following reperfusion as the result of PCI are similar to the improvements seen with successful pharmacologic reperfusion, but slightly better in many studies. Most of the benefits of PCI over thrombolytic therapy, however, come from reductions in late reinfarctions. Data suggesting greater acute salvage of muscle with PCI as compared to thrombolysis are not as clear.

When PCI is utilized as the initial therapeutic strategy for STEMI it is called *primary PCI*. However, in those situations where primary PCI is not available within 90 min and patients receive thrombolytic therapy, patients are often referred for emergent PCI if they do not demonstrate evidence of reperfusion within 30–60 min of administration of the fibrinolytic drug. PCI in this instance is called *rescue PCI*.

Components of Delay in Implementing Reperfusion Strategies

The total elapsed time from the onset of symptoms to administration of a thrombolytic agent, or to PCI, can be divided into three distinct phases. The first phase is the time required for the patient to recognize that something is wrong and make the decision to access the medical system. The second is the time required for the prehospital emergency medical system to respond, render emergency care, and transport the patient to a medical facility. The third phase consists of the time required for the hospital to recognize AMI, qualify the patient, and implement either pharmacologic thrombolysis or PCI.

Phase 1 is beyond the direct control of medical personnel. Efforts to impact the first phase through programs of public education have been disappointing. The second and third phases, however, are within the direct control of the medical community. Reducing times to reperfusion requires a coordinated effort between prehospital and hospital personnel and the establishment of clear protocols for the evaluation and treatment of patients with chest pain.

Reducing Times to Reperfusion

Prehospital Protocols

The effort to speed reperfusion should begin with the prehospital emergency medical system. Multiple studies have now clearly demonstrated that in-hospital times to thrombolysis are significantly reduced by the performance of a prehospital ECG.[18-21] Prehospital ACLS providers have readily mastered the technique of performing an ECG, and on-scene times have been minimally impacted by this additional task, increasing by only 2–5 min.

Interpretation of the ECG can be accomplished by cellular or satellite telemetry to a physician at the base hospital, by computer interpretation, or by independent sight-reading of the tracing by trained prehospital ACLS providers. The hospital emergency department is then notified by radio that a prequalified potential candidate for reperfusion is en route. The ability of the hospital team to "gear-up" based on such field reports has been reported to save from 29 to 71 min in-hospital.[18-21]

Other necessary, but time-consuming, elements of every reperfusion protocol, such as drawing blood, starting intravenous lines, and administering aspirin, can also often be partially or completely accomplished en route. The prehospital provider can also continue to converse with the patient during the above procedures and complete the initial screen for contraindications to thrombolysis.

Finally, ACC/AHA guidelines also recommend prehospital administration of aspirin (chewed) to patients suspected of having STEMI, unless there are contraindications to aspirin, such as aspirin allergy.[12]

Prehospital Fibrinolysis

Some high-performance ACLS units have successfully implemented protocols for prehospital thrombolysis in a further effort to reduce times to reperfusion. Studies have shown reductions in time to thrombolysis ranging from 28 to 73 min, depending on whether patient calls originated in metropolitan or rural locations.[22] In the CAPTIM trial there was a strong trend toward lower mortality and a reduction in cardiogenic shock with prehospital fibrinolysis (mean time 130 min from onset of symptoms) versus PCI (mean time 190 min from onset of symptoms).[23]

ACC/AHA guidelines assert that such a protocol of prehospital fibrinolysis is reasonable in 1) settings in which physicians are present in the ambulance or 2) well-organized EMS systems with full-time paramedics who have 12-lead ECGs in the field with transmission capability, paramedic initial and ongoing training in ECG interpretation and STEMI treatment, online medical command, a medical director with training/experience in STEMI management, and an ongoing continuous quality-improvement program.[12]

In-Hospital Protocols

Elapsed times from patient arrival to initiation of reperfusion therapy at the hospital cannot be reduced without two key hospital policies that have been agreed upon by the medical staff. The first is that hospital emergency department physicians must have the ability to initiate thrombolytic therapy or make arrangements for PCI on their own authority. Waiting for an evaluation by a consulting cardiologist is one of the biggest sources of in-hospital delay.

The second key policy is that in those instances where thrombolytic therapy is chosen, it must be initiated in the emergency department as opposed to waiting until the patient is transferred to the coronary care unit.

With these two key policies in place, the emergency department can proceed to establish effective protocols for speeding reperfusion therapy.

Emergency department protocols for dealing with potential reperfusion candidates should be the equivalent of a major trauma plan and carry the same sense of urgency. The following are essential components of an effective protocol:

1. The protocol must be in writing, including drug preparation instructions and dosage charts, and conveniently posted in appropriate locations.
2. Nursing triage staff must have the ability to initiate the protocol before the patient has been seen by the physician, including starting IVs, drawing blood, and performing a 12-lead ECG, particularly on patients who do not arrive via the emergency medical system.

3. All necessary supplies and medications for fibrinolytic therapy should be kept in a kit or single, readily accessible location.
4. Minimum mandatory criteria necessary for emergency department physicians to initiate thrombolytic therapy should be confined to a history, physical examination, and ECG compatible with AMI. Therapy should not be delayed awaiting laboratory results.

The goal of such organizational efforts should be to administer fibrinolytic therapy to appropriate candidates within <30 min from the time of arrival in the emergency department or to accomplish PCI in <90 min. A few institutions have been successful in routinely accomplishing initiation of therapy in <15 min when the presentation of STEMI is straightforward.

Treatment of NSTEMI

A high percentage of patients with both unstable angina and NSTEMI have been demonstrated to have a nonocclusive thrombus growing on a ruptured atherosclerotic plaque. In many of these patients, the elevation of biochemical markers (cardiac enzymes) is believed to be caused by microembolization of platelet aggregates and components of the disrupted plaque into the microvasculature of the myocardium distal to the lesion.

Despite the evidence of a thrombotic etiology, fibrinolytic therapy has, counterintuitively, clearly been shown to provide no benefit, and in some studies actually increased the risk of subsequent infarction. Therapy for unstable angina/NSTEMI is therefore directed primarily at inhibiting platelet aggregation and inhibiting the coagulation cascade so as to prevent further propagation of the nonocclusive clot.

The mainstay of treatment is aspirin, clopidogrel (Plavix), and IIb/IIIa inhibitors aimed at inhibiting platelet aggregation; unfractionated heparin or low molecular weight heparin to inhibit the coagulation cascade; and other standard drugs to treat ischemia, including nitrates and beta blockers.

Risk stratification and decisions to move to angiography and PCI are sometimes difficult and beyond the scope of this text. Said decisions, however, are not frequently the province of the ACLS provider.

References

1. DeWood MA, Spores J, Notske R, et al. Prevalence of total coronary artery occlusion during the early hours of transmural myocardial infarction. *N Engl J Med.* 1980;303:897–902.
2. Hochman JS, Sleeper LA, White HD, et al. For the Should We Emergently Revascularize Occluded Coronaries for Cardiogenic Shock (SHOCK) Investigators. One-year survival following early revascularization for cardiogenic shock. *JAMA.* 2001;285:190–192.
3. Hochman JS, Sleeper LA, Webb JG, et al. For the Should We Emergently Revascularize Occluded Coronaries for Cardiogenic Shock (SHOCK) Investigators. Early revascularization in acute myocardial infarction complicated by cardiogenic shock. *N Engl J Med* 1999;341:625–634.
4. Cerqueirs M, Litwin P, Martin J, et al. Infarct size reduction and preservation of ejection fraction with very early thrombolytic treatment for myocardial

infarction; radionuclide results from the Myocardial Infarction Triage and Inter-vention Trial. [Abstract]. *Circulation*. 1992;86:643.

5. Gruppo Italiano per lo Studio della Streptochi-nasi nell'Infarto Miocardico (GISSI). Long-term effects of intravenous thrombolysis in acute myocardial infarction: a final report of the GISSI study. *Lancet*. 1987;2:871–874.

6. Koren G, Weiss AT, Hasin Y, et al. Prevention of myocardial damage in acute myocardial ischemia by early treatment with intravenous streptokinase. *N Engl J Med*. 1985;313:1384–1389.

7. Fine DG, Weiss AT, Sapoznikov D, et al. Importance of early initiation of intra-venous streptokinase therapy for acute myocardial infarction. *Am J Cardiol*. 1986;58:411–417.

8. Gruppo Italiano per lo Studio della Streptochi-nasi nell'Infarto Miocardico (GISSI). Effectiveness of intravenous thrombolytic treatment in acute myocardial infarction. *Lancet*. 1986;1:397.

9. ISIS-2. Randomized trial of intravenous streptokinase, oral aspirin, both, or neither among 17,187 cases of suspected acute myocardial infarction: ISIS-2. ISIS-2 (Second International Study of Infarct Survival) Collaborative Group. *Lancet*. 1988;2(8607):349–360.

10. ISIS-3. A randomized comparison of streptokinase vs tissue plasminogen acti-vator vs anistreplase and of aspirin plus heparin vs aspirin alone among 41,299 cases of suspected acute myocardial infarction. ISIS-3 (Third International Study of Infarct Survival) Collaborative Group. *Lancet*. 1992;339(8796):753–770.

11. LATE Study Group. Late Assessment of Thrombolytic Efficacy (LATE) study with alteplase 6–24 hours after onset of acute myocardial infarction. Lancet 1993;342(8874):759–766.

12. Antman EM, Anbe DT, Armstrong PW, et al. ACC/AHA Guidelines for the Management of Patients With ST-Elevation Myocardial Infarction: A report of the American College of Cardiology/American Heart Association Task Force on Practice Guidelines (Committee to Revise the 1999 Guidelines for the Management of Patients With Acute Myocardial Infarction). Available at www.acc.org/clinical/guidelines/stemi/guideline/index.htm.

13. Tiefenbrunn AJ, Sobel BE. The impact of coronary thrombolysis on myocardial infarction. *Fibrinolysis*. 1989;3:1–15.

14. GISSI-2. A factorial randomized trial of alteplase versus streptokinase and heparin versus no heparin among 12,490 patients with acute myocardial infarc-tion. *Lancet*. 1990;336:65–71.

15. GUSTO. An international randomized trial comparing four thrombolytic strate-gies for acute myocardial infarction. The GUSTO investigators. *N Eng J Med*. 1993;329(10):723–725.

16. Tiefenbrunn AJ, Ludbrook PA. Coronary thrombolysis- it's worth the risk. *JAMA*. 1989;261:2107.

17. Lange RA, Hillis LD. Immediate angioplasty for acute myocardial infarction. *N Eng J Med*. 1993;328(10):726–728.

18. Karagounis L, Ipsen SK, Jessop MR, et al. Impact of field-transmitted electrocar-diography on time to in-hospital thrombolytic therapy in acute myocardial infarction. *Am J Cardiol*. 1990;66:786–791.

19. Gibler WB, Kereiakes DJ, Dean EN, et al. Prehospital diagnosis and treatment of acute myocardial infarction: a north-south perspective. *Am Heart J*. 1991;121: 1–11.

20. Kennedy JW, Weaver WD. The potential for prehospital thrombolytic therapy. *Clin Cardiol*. 1990;13:VIII23–26.

21. Foster DB, Dufendach JH, Barkdoll CM, et al. Prehospital recognition of AMI using independent nurse/paramedic 12-lead ECG evaluation: impact on in-hospital times to thrombolysis in a rural community hospital. *Am J Emerg Med*. 1994;1:25–31.

22. Pedley DK, Bissett K, Connolly EM, et al. Prospective observational cohort study of time saved by prehospital thrombolysis for ST elevation myocardial infarction delivered by paramedics. *BMJ*. 2003;327:22–26.

23. Bonnefoy E, Lapostolle F, Leizorovicz A, et al. Primary angioplasty versus prehospital fibrinolysis in acute myocardial infarction: a randomized study. *Lancet*. 2002;360:825–829.

13

Miscellaneous Conditions

In this final chapter, we will discuss a potpourri of essentially unrelated medical conditions that can sometimes produce dramatic changes in the appearance of the ECG.

Electrolyte Disturbances

Alterations in certain serum electrolytes, particularly in serum potassium and calcium, can produce rather dramatic changes in the ECG because of their roles in membrane repolarization and depolarization. As you will recall, influx and efflux of positive ions across cell membranes are the basis for the electrical activity of cells. Alterations in their concentrations could be expected to change the behavior of that electrical activity, and therefore, to also change the ECG.

Hypokalemia

When serum potassium concentrations fall below approximately 3.0 mEq/L, ST segments begin to sag, T waves begin to flatten or invert, and U waves begin to become more prominent, sometimes exceeding the T wave in height. Often, the flattened T wave and the prominent U wave begin to merge, giving the false appearance of a prolonged QT interval. Figure 13.1 illustrates these hallmarks of hypokalemia. Note that the take-off, or J point, of the ST segment is depressed. The net effect of these changes is a rather undulating appearance to the combined ST segment, T wave, and U wave.

Patients with hypokalemia are more prone to life-threatening ventricular dysrhythmias, particularly when on digitalis preparations. Common clinical conditions predisposing to hypokalemia include diuretic administration and vomiting (hypochloremic alkalosis), and correction of diabetic ketoacidosis without adequate potassium replacement.

Figure 13.1. Leads V₄–V₆ from a patient with a serum potassium of 2.6. Note J point depression and a sagging ST segment. The flattened T waves and prominent U waves have almost merged to give the false appearance of a prolonged QT interval.

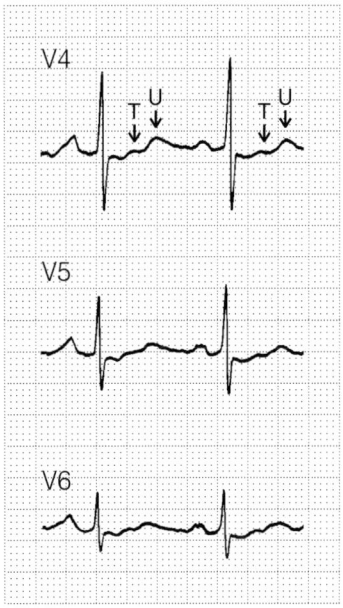

Hyperkalemia

Many of the ECG changes seen with hyperkalemia are simply the opposite of those seen with hypokalemia. As serum potassium levels begin to rise above approximately 5.5 mEq/L, T waves become very tall and peaked (Figure 13.2). J-point ST elevation may occur, simulating AMI. Further elevations in

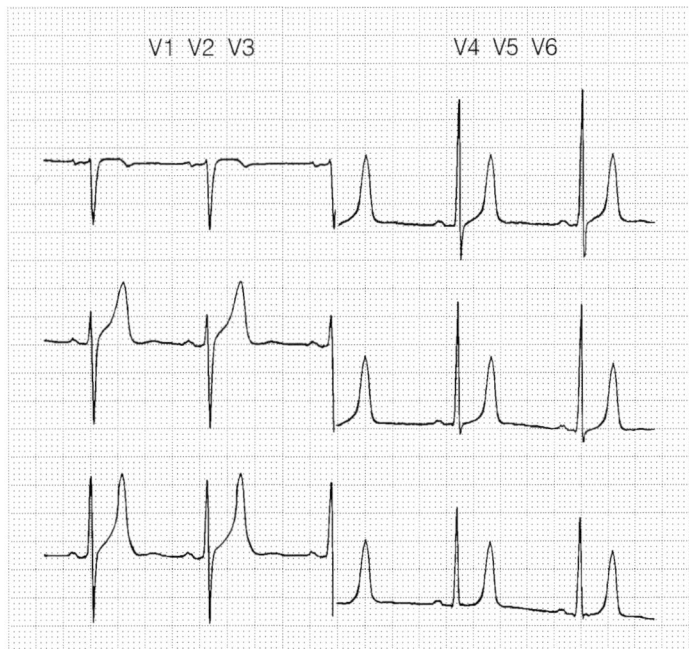

Figure 13.2. ECG changes associated with moderate hyperkalemia. Note that T waves are tall and symmetrically peaked, and that there is mild J point elevation in V₂ and V₃.

potassium begin to produce lengthening PR intervals and nonspecific, but often dramatic, QRS widening. P waves begin to flatten and may disappear altogether. The terminal event is asystole or ventricular fibrillation.

Figure 13.3A is the ECG of a 52-year-old white male seen in the emergency department with a serum potassium of 8.1 mEq/L on the basis of renal failure and diabetic ketoacidosis. Note that P waves cannot be seen in most leads, and there is diffuse nonspecific widening of the QRS to over 0.20 s. Figure 13.3B is a tracing taken on the same patient after treatment with intravenous calcium gluconate, bicarbonate, and insulin. Note that although clear P waves

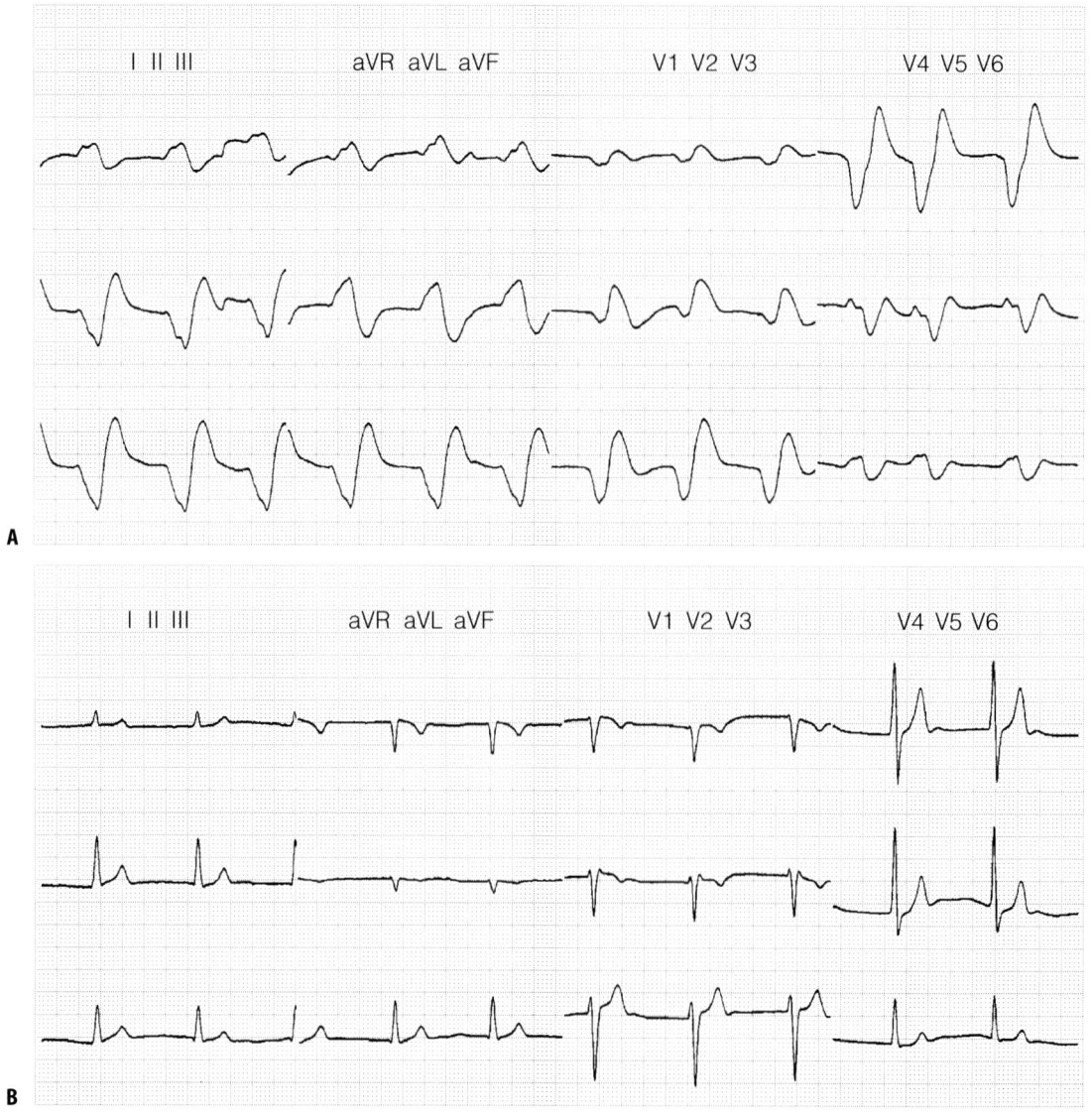

Figure 13.3 A. Severe hyperkalemia. ECG of a 52-year-old white male with renal failure and diabetic ketoacidosis, and a serum potassium of 8.1. P waves are absent, and the QRS is widened to over 0.20 s. **B.** ECG of the same patient as in Figure 13.3A, but after treatment with IV calcium gluconate, insulin, and sodium bicarbonate.

have not yet returned, the QRS has dramatically narrowed, and T waves in V_4 and V_5 have taken on the tall, peaked appearance typical of lower levels of hyperkalemia.

As with hypokalemia, ventricular fibrillation may be the ultimate consequence of progressive hyperkalemia. Common causes of hyperkalemia include renal failure, acidosis, administration of aldosterone antagonists, and administration of exogenous potassium.

Hypocalcemia

The hallmark of hypocalcemia is a prolonged QT interval. Occasionally T wave inversion will also occur, but this is unusual. Clinically significant hypocalcemia is rare, and the primary cause is usually hypoparathyroidism.

Hypercalcemia

Elevations of serum calcium produce the opposite to those produced by hypocalcemia, namely a shortened QT interval, often with a very abrupt upslope of the T wave.

Hypercalcemia is more common than hypocalcemia. Major causes include advanced malignancy, hyperparathyroidism, and sarcoidosis.

Drug-Induced ECG Changes

Several drugs can produce changes in the ECG, but the most important are *digitalis, quinidine,* and *procainamide.* The changes induced by these drugs, although sometimes characteristic, are often nonspecific, and are easily confused with other causes of ECG abnormalities.

The primary usefulness in recognizing the abnormalities that can be caused by drugs is to rule out a drug-induced etiology for various ECG findings before concluding that they are the result of primary myocardial disease. In addition, a familiarity with drug-induced ECG changes can aid in suspecting drug toxicity when ECG changes occur acutely in patients on these drugs.

Digitalis Effect

Digitalis products, even in therapeutic, nontoxic doses, can produce sagging of the ST segment, flattening of T waves, and shortening of the QT interval. The ST depression is upwardly concave, as opposed to its appearance in LVH, for instance, which is upwardly convex. Figure 13.4 shows these typical changes in the ECG of a patient with therapeutic levels of digoxin.

Digitalis intoxication can produce multiple rhythm disturbances, including the classic junctional tachycardia, paroxysmal atrial tachycardia with block, all forms of ventricular ectopy, and all forms of heart block.

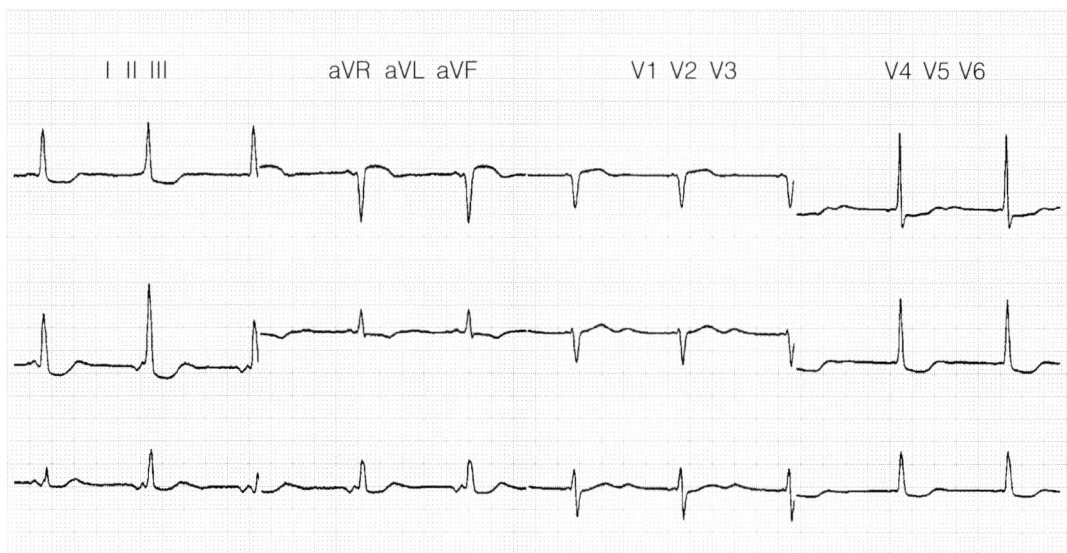

I II III　　　　aVR aVL aVF　　　　V1 V2 V3　　　　V4 V5 V6

Figure 13.4. Typically sagging ST segments of digitalis effect. Note that the patient is in a junctional rhythm.

Quinidine Effect

The primary effect of quinidine is on T waves and the QT interval. T waves become widened, flattened, and ultimately inverted. Marked lengthening of the QT interval can occur and can contribute to the proarrhythmic effect sometimes noted with quinidine. In addition, significant widening of the QRS occurs at toxic levels.

Figure 13.5 shows the precordial leads of a 75-year-old white female who had recently been started on quinidine for atrial fibrillation. This tracing

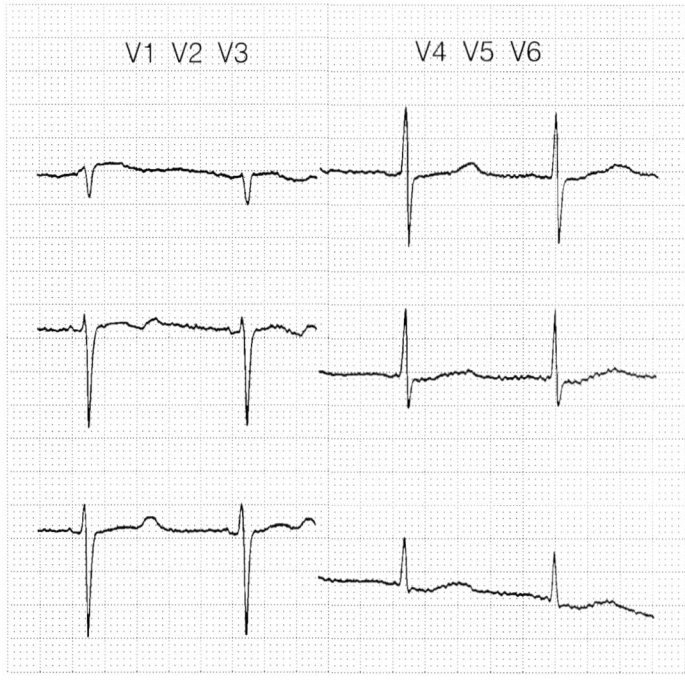

V1 V2 V3　　　　V4 V5 V6

Figure 13.5. Precordial leads of a 75-year-old white female on quinidine just after cardioversion from ventricular fibrillation. Note the prolonged QT interval and the flattening and widening of T waves. Considerable muscle artifact is present.

was taken just minutes after conversion from an episode of ventricular fibrillation precipitated by the proarrhythmic effect of quinidine. Note that the QT interval is prolonged and that the T waves are flattened and widened.

Procainamide Effect

The primary effect of procaineamide is widening of the QRS at toxic doses. An increase in QRS duration of 50% or more is one of the endpoints for procainamide administration.

Intracranial Hemorrhage

Cerebral hemorrhage or other causes of rapid rises in intracranial pressure can produce bradycardia, widening of the T waves, and T wave inversion across the precordial leads. Such changes are an ominous prognostic sign. Figure 13.6 shows the tracing of an elderly white female with an ultimately fatal extensive cerebral hemorrhage.

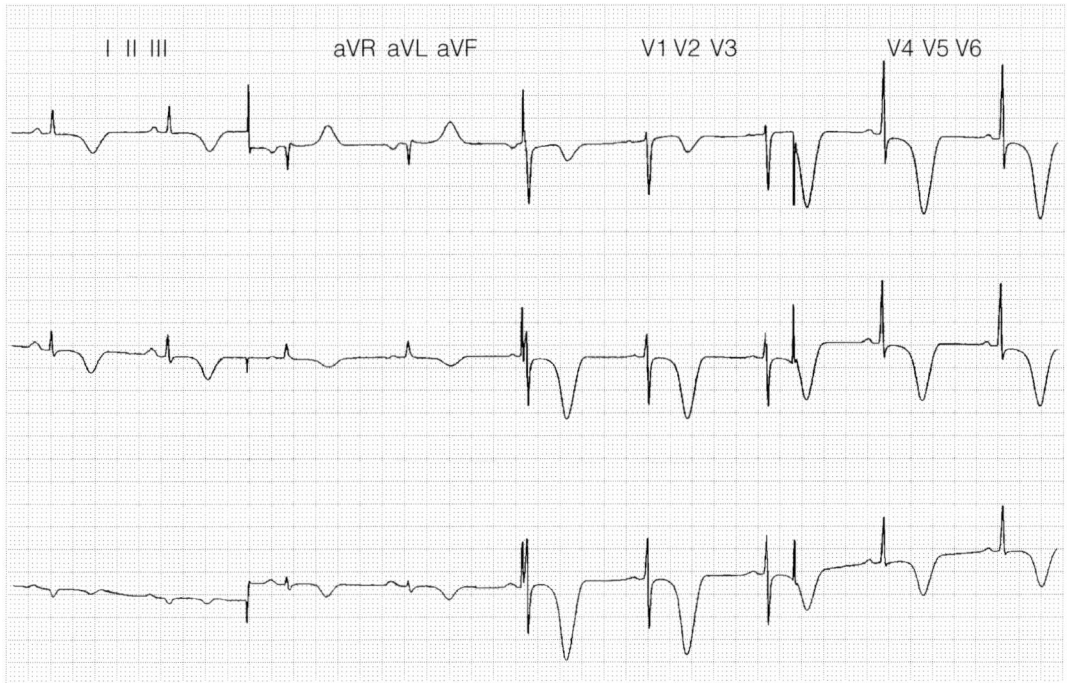

Figure 13.6. ECG tracing just before death of an elderly white female with a massive cerebral hemorrhage. Note the deep, symmetrical T wave inversion, particularly across the precordial leads.

Diffuse Low Voltage

Low voltage throughout the 12-lead ECG can be seen with hypothyroidism, pericardial effusion, and diffuse cardiomyopathy of ischemic or other origin.

Pericarditis

The ECG changes of acute pericarditis, like those of AMI, go through an evolutionary process over a period of weeks. But, as you will recall from the discussion of the differential diagnoses of ST elevation in Chapter 9, there are significant differences that usually permit us to distinguish between the two.

ST elevation is the usual initial hallmark of both pericarditis and AMI. The ST elevation of pericarditis, however, is usually upwardly concave, widespread throughout all leads, and without reciprocal ST depression.

T wave inversion follows ST elevation as the ST segments return to baseline, but the Q waves seen with AMI never develop.

Another interesting and unique finding with pericarditis is depression of the PR segment. Figure 13.7 is the ECG of a 37-year-old white male with acute viral pericarditis. Note that the PR segments are depressed below the baseline and that there is widespread, upwardly concave ST elevation, without reciprocal depression and without Q wave formation.

Acute pericarditis often undergoes ECG evolution, much as does AMI, except for Q wave formation, which does not occur with pericarditis. ST-segment elevation will show resolution, however, and, as with AMI, T waves may invert.

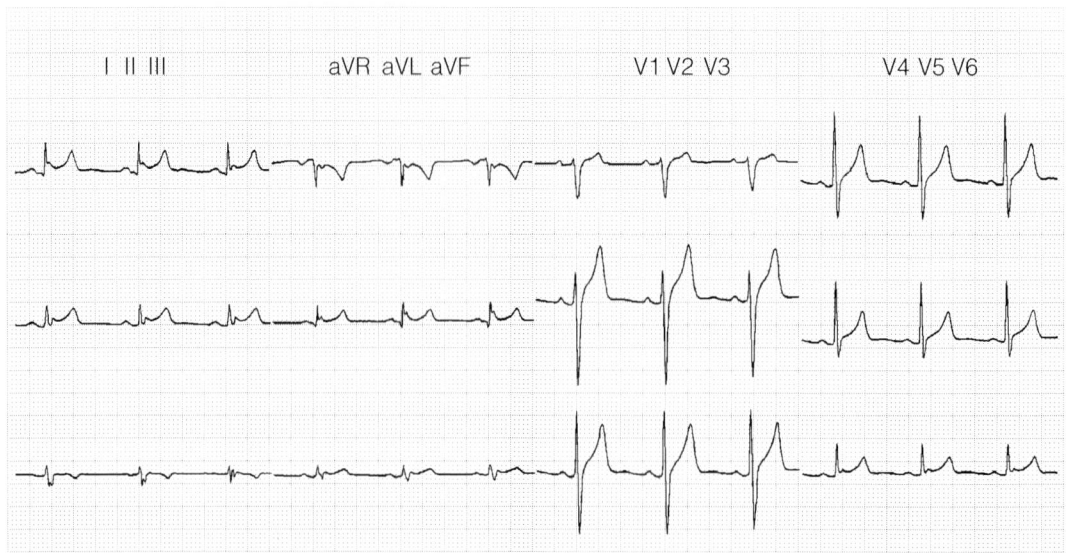

Figure 13.7. Acute viral pericarditis in a 37-year-old white male. Note the widespread, upwardly concave ST elevation, depressed PR segment, and absence of Q waves or reciprocal depression.

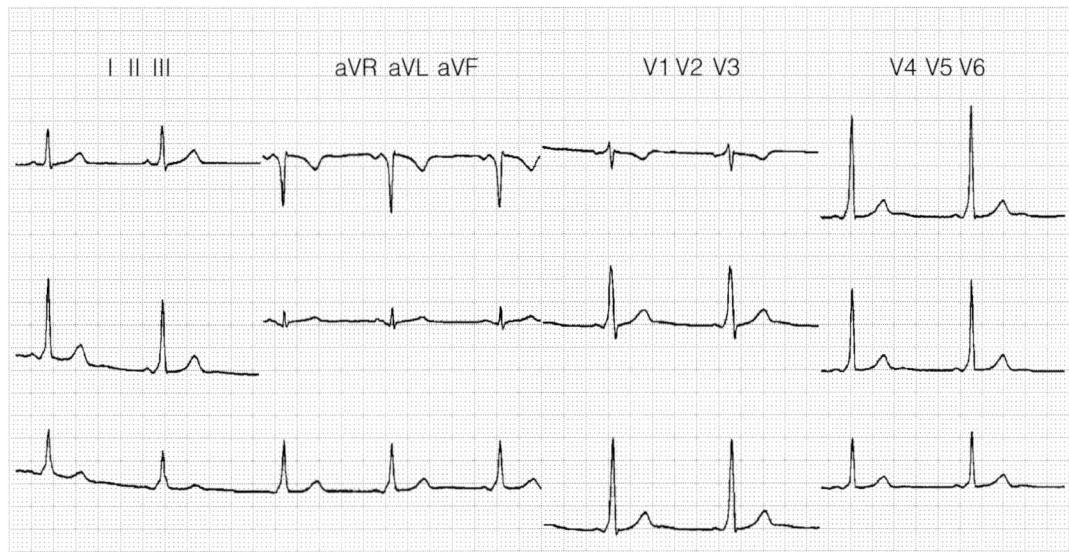

Figure 13.8. WPW syndrome with a short PR interval, and delta waves seen in most leads.

Wolff–Parkinson–White Syndrome

Wolff–Parkinson–White syndrome is the result of a congenital *accessory pathway* to the ventricles that bypasses the AV node, resulting in *preexcitation* of the ventricles. The impulse still goes down through the AV node normally, but also goes down the accessory pathway, which conducts much faster than the AV node. The result is that the impulse gets to the ventricles early via the accessory pathway, producing an early slurred upstroke of the R wave called a *delta wave* (Figure 2.4).

This early delta wave also produces a short PR interval and widening of the QRS. Often, however, the remainder of the QRS after the delta wave looks normal because, in many instances, most of the ventricular muscle is still depolarized via the normal conduction system. In other cases, a large amount of muscle may be depolarized by slow muscle-to-muscle conduction initiated by the accessory pathway and may produce a QRS, an ST segment, and T waves looking more like a BBB pattern.

Figure 13.8 is the tracing of a 44-year-old white male with a history of WPW syndrome. Note that the PR interval is short and there is a clear delta wave seen in most, but not all, leads. In the case of this particular patient, the remainder of the QRS looks normal.

Hypothermia

Marked hypothermia produces prominent bradycardia, first degree AV block, and QRS abnormalities at the J point (junction of the QRS and ST segment) called *J waves* or *Osborn waves*. Characteristically, there is J point elevation, and the Osborn wave then slopes down over approximately 0.04 s into the ST segment.

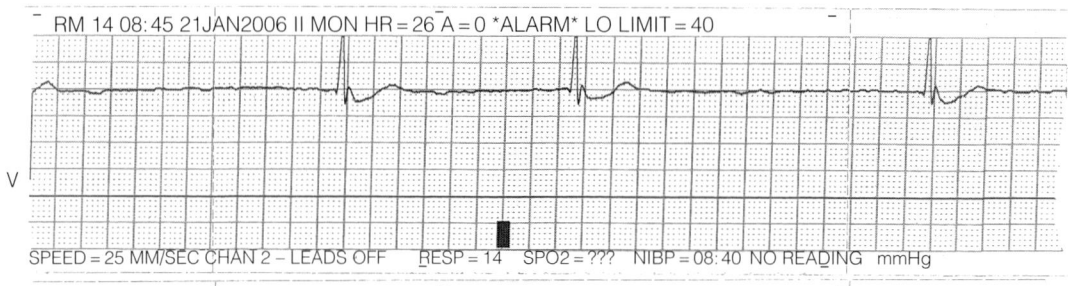

Figure 13.9. Osborne waves or J waves associated with a core body temperature of 84.6°F in a 32-year-old male heroin overdose patient suffering from exposure. Note that the rate is slow, P waves are difficult to identify, and there is J-point elevation, with the Osborne wave then sloping down into the ST segment over about 0.04 s.

Figure 13.9 shows a rhythm strip from a 32-year-old male who presented with a heroin overdose after being outside all night. His core body temperature at admission was 84.6 degrees Fahrenheit. P waves are of low amplitude and difficult to discern. Osborn waves are prominently visible as shown by the arrow. Figure 13.10 is the full 12-lead tracing after substantial rewarming. Heart rate has increased and P waves are now more visible, but first-degree heart block remains, and prominent J waves are still present.

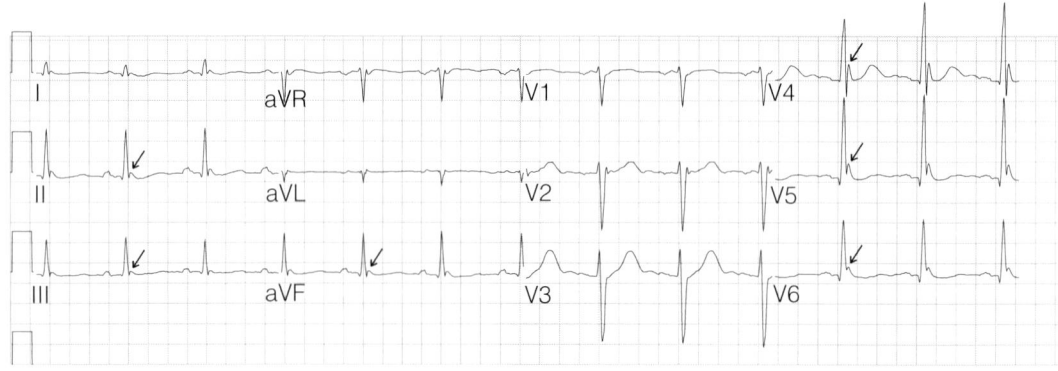

Figure 13.10. Twelve-lead ECG of the same patient after substantial rewarming. Note that the P waves are now quite visible, but J waves remain, although they are less prominent than in Figure 13.9.

14

Case Presentations

This section is designed to give you some practice in implementing your newfound knowledge in making clinical decisions regarding the patient with a potential acute coronary syndrome, much as ACLS megacodes permit you to practice resuscitation. There are 12 practice case presentations. You will have the opportunity to make decisions in a sequential fashion, much as you would do in real-life clinical situations. Sometimes you will be functioning in the prehospital environment, and sometimes in the emergency department or coronary care unit. For purposes of this section you should assume that the phrase *prehospital thrombolytic protocol* refers to (1) starting two IVs, (2) drawing blood specimens for laboratory analysis in the process of starting the IVs, and (3) administering one aspirin to be chewed—all of these in preparation for potential thrombolysis in the emergency department.

Because a decision to implement thrombolysis is often more complex than a decision to refer the patient to an interventional cardiologist for emergent PCI, most of the following scenarios that involve a patient with STEMI assume that interventional cardiology is not immediately available, or is too far away to warrant the diversion of an ambulance.

Policies regarding the authority of individual paramedics, nurses, and even physicians to initiate procedures or therapy vary from jurisdiction to jurisdiction. Assume for the purposes of this section that you always have the authority to proceed without consulting a higher authority when presented with diagnostic or therapeutic options. You should find it to be fun.

Case 1

You are functioning as a prehospital ACLS provider today in a community more than 2 hours away from the closest cardiac catheterization facility. Acute STEMIs are therefore treated in your local hospital with thrombolytics. You are dispatched to a local accounting firm to help a 39-year-old black male with a chief complaint of retrosternal chest discomfort with minimal radiation to the left shoulder. The pain came on while he was sitting at his desk, is described as a pressure, and has been present for a little over 3 hours. He admits to mild nausea, but denies vomiting, diaphoresis, or shortness of breath. He has not tried antacids or nitroglycerin for relief. He awoke with a similar discomfort about three nights ago, went into the bathroom and got a drink, and then lay down and fell asleep again. He has had no exertional chest discomfort with exercise such as mowing the lawn with a push lawnmower.

He has been told in the past that his blood pressure was "a little high," but no medications were prescribed. He smokes one pack of cigarettes daily. His father died quite suddenly in his early 50s.

Physical examination reveals a mildly obese black male who appears anxious. Pulse, 80. Respirations, 20. BP, 184/112. His skin is warm and dry. He has no jugular venous distention. The lungs are clear. Hearth rhythm is regular, and the heart tones are not muffled. You can hear no gallop, murmurs, or friction rubs. He has no peripheral edema.

1. With regard to the pain, you conclude that:
   a) the history is sufficient to be compatible with ACS.
   b) the history is not compatible with ACS.
2. With regard to the physical examination, you conclude that:
   a) the physical examination lends support to the diagnosis of ACS.
   b) the physical examination neither confirms nor denies the possibility of ACS.
3. Your first procedural step should be to:
   a) give 0.4 mg sublingual nitroglycerin.
   b) start a medical IV, attach the patient to a cardiac monitor, and start O_2.
   c) perform a 12-lead electrocardiogram.
   d) question the patient regarding contraindications to thrombolytic therapy.
4. Your second procedural step should be to:
   a) give 0.4 mg sublingual nitroglycerin.
   b) start a medical IV, attach the patient to a cardiac monitor, and start O_2.
   c) perform a 12-lead electrocardiogram.
   d) question the patient regarding contraindications to thrombolytic therapy.
5. Your third procedural step should be to:
   a) give 0.4 mg sublingual nitroglycerin.
   b) start a medical IV, attach the patient to a cardiac monitor, start O_2.
   c) perform a 12-lead electrocardiogram.
   d) question the patient regarding contraindications to thrombolytic therapy.

You have performed a 12-lead ECG (Figure 14.1). Questioning conducted during performance of the ECG revealed that the patient had a hernia repair 2 years ago. He admits to an allergy to aspirin and states that he breaks out in hives when he takes the drug.

6. Upon completion of the ECG, you quickly note that the patient's electrocardiogram shows:
   a) a normal axis.
   b) RAD.

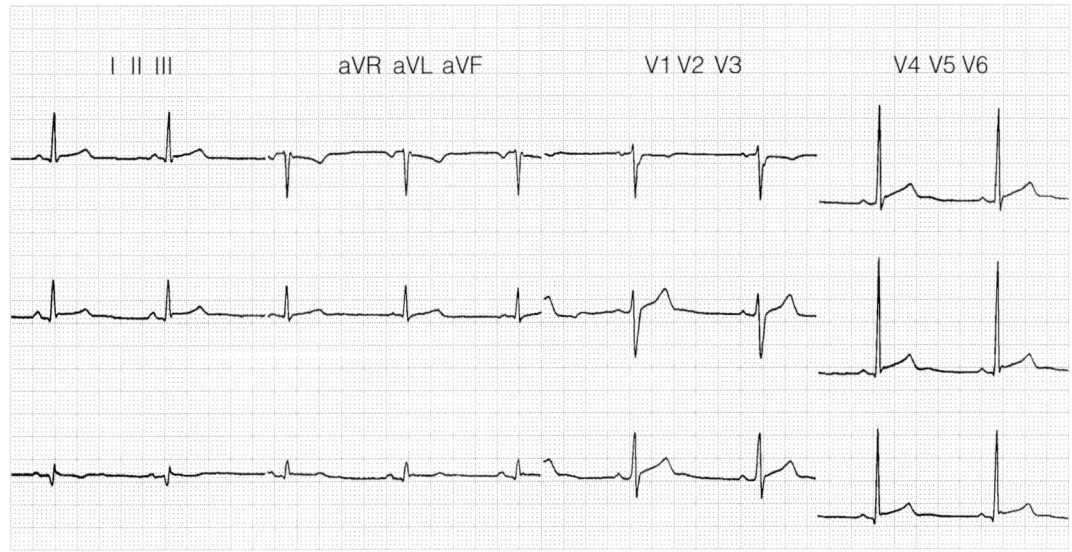

Figure 14.1.

   c) LAD.
   d) an indeterminate axis.
7. With regard to contraindications to aspirin, you conclude that:
   a) contraindications exist.
   b) no contraindications exist.
8. With regard to contraindications to thrombolytic agents, on the basis of currently available information you conclude that:
   a) absolute contraindications exist.
   b) relative contraindications exist.
   c) no contraindications exist.
9. Upon contacting medical command by radio, you report that the ECG shows:
   a) an acute inferior STEMI.
   b) an acute anterior STEMI.
   c) an inferior myocardial infarction that may be old.
   d) an anterior myocardial infarction that may be old.
   e) benign early repolarization changes.
   f) a LBBB simulating anterior STEMI.
   g) acute pericarditis.
   h) a normal ECG.
   i) nonspecific ST changes.
10. Your field assessment, as reported to medical command, is that:
   a) sufficient evidence of STEMI exists to recommend thrombolytic therapy and to institute the prehospital thrombolytic protocol.
   b) sufficient evidence of STEMI exists to recommend thrombolytic therapy with the exception of aspirin, if relative contraindications can be removed.
   c) evidence of STEMI exists, but absolute contraindications prohibit thrombolytic therapy.

d) evidence of STEMI exists, but relative contraindications rule out thrombolytic therapy.

e) Insufficient evidence of STEMI exists to recommend either thrombolytic therapy or implementation of the prehospital thrombolytic protocol.

f) Insufficient evidence of STEMI exists to recommend thrombolytic therapy at present, but the index of suspicion is still high enough to warrant implementation of the prehospital thrombolytic protocol, with the exception of aspirin.

Answers and Case Discussion

1. a   2. b   3. b   4. c   5. a   6. a   7. a   8. b   9. e   10. f

This 39-year-old man had the significant risk factors of a family history of cardiovascular disease, cigarette smoking, and hypertension. Although vomiting, diaphoresis, and shortness of breath were not present, his history is still compatible with AMI. The physical examination is not helpful in this instance and neither confirms nor denies the possibility of AMI. As always, the first steps to be taken should be those that are necessary to protect the patient's life should an adverse event such as ventricular fibrillation occur. Therefore, starting an IV, monitoring the patient, and starting O_2 are the first steps.

Because administration of nitroglycerin could cause resolution of important diagnostic changes on the ECG, such as ST elevation or depression, the ECG should be performed before nitroglycerin is administered. Little harm is done by delaying nitroglycerin for the several minutes required to do the ECG, and you may prevent the patient from facing the possibility of an inconclusive diagnosis that would have been clear if the ECG had been done first.

The ECG tracing shows a normal axis of approximately 30 degrees. ST elevation, which is upwardly concave, is widespread in all walls of the heart. There is no reciprocal depression. A small Q is present in lead III, but it is not pathologic, and there is no pathologic Q present in adjacent lead aVF. There is no PR-segment depression, as is often seen in pericarditis. Therefore, benign early repolarization changes are the most likely source of the ST-segment elevation, although pericarditis is still possible.

The patient's current hypertension provides a relative contraindication to thrombolytic agents, although one could still be administered if the projected benefit outweighed the risk or if treatment was administered and resulted in the BP falling below 180/110. Aspirin is, of course, absolutely contraindicated because of the clear history of allergy, and in this case, one might want to use clopidogrel.

We are, thus, left with a patient with significant risk factors and a history compatible with AMI, who has a contraindication to aspirin and a relative contraindication to thrombolytics. His ECG is not compatible with AMI at the present time. Nevertheless, his history is compatible with AMI, and it is quite possible that a repeat ECG upon arrival at the hospital might show AMI. Therefore, there is insufficient evidence of STEMI to recommend him for thrombolytic therapy, but it is probably best to place him in a category of "negative ECG, but high index of suspicion" and to draw blood and start two IVs while en route to the hospital.

Case 2

You are functioning as an emergency department physician. It is 10:15 PM. The nurses ask you to see a 52-year-old white female with a chief complaint of epigastric and lower retrosternal "indigestion" that radiates through to between her shoulder blades. The pain came on at approximately 6:45 PM, shortly after a supper of ham and potatoes. She has never had a similar pain. She admits to nausea, and she vomited one time shortly after dinner. Her blouse became damp with perspiration after vomiting. She feels mildly short of breath. She tried a half teaspoon of baking soda in half a glass of water to relieve the indigestion, but got no relief.

The patient carries a history of hypertension and diabetes. She is taking Lopressor 50 mg bid, and an oral hypoglycemic. There is no history of tobacco use. She has no knowledge of what her cholesterol level might be. Her father died of a stroke in his 70 s, and her mother died of heart failure, also in her 70 s, but she can think of no one in the family who ever had a heart attack.

Physical examination reveals an obese white female who appears uncomfortable. Pulse, 75. Respirations, 22. BP, 190/114. Her skin is warm, but damp. She has no jugular venous distension. The lungs are clear. Heart rhythm is regular, and an S_4 gallop is audible. Her abdomen is soft and not really tender, but it makes her feel sick to the stomach when you palpate the epigastrium. She has no peripheral edema.

1. With regard to the pain, you conclude that:
   a) the history is adequate to be compatible with AMI.
   b) the history is not compatible with AMI.
2. With regard to the physical examination, you conclude that:
   a) the physical exam lends support to the diagnosis of AMI.
   b) the physical exam neither confirms nor denies the possibility of AMI.

The nursing staff has already started O_2 at 4L by nasal cannula, and has attached the patient to a cardiac monitor, noninvasive BP machine, and pulse oximeter.

3. Your first procedural step should be to:
   a) order 0.4 mg sublingual nitroglycerin.
   b) order a medical IV.
   c) perform a stat 12-ead electrocardiogram.
   d) order appropriate bloodworm.
   e) order a gallbladder sonogram.
4. Your second procedural step should be to:
   a) order 0.4 mg sublingual nitroglycerin.
   b) order a medical IV.
   c) perform a stat 12-lead electrocardiogram.
   d) order appropriate bloodwork.
   e) order a gallbladder sonogram.

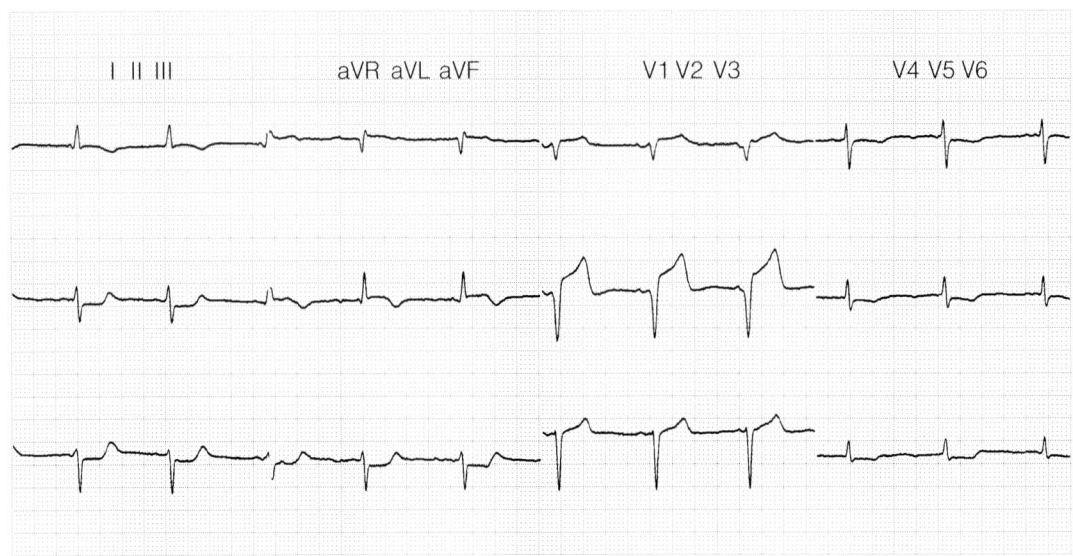

Figure 14.2.

A 12-lead ECG has been performed (Figure 14.2). Questioning conducted during performance of the ECG reveals that the patient has no known allergies, has had only one hospitalization, other than childbirth, for a hysterectomy 3 years ago, and has no other chronic illnesses and no history of significant injury.

5. Upon completion of the ECG, you quickly note that the patient's electrocardiogram shows:
   a) a normal axis.
   b) RAD.
   c) LAD.
   d) an indeterminate axis.
6. On the basis of currently available information, you conclude that thrombolytic agents, if necessary, would be:
   a) absolutely contraindicated.
   b) relatively contraindicated.
   c) not contraindicated.
7. With regard to contraindications to aspirin, should it be necessary, you conclude that:
   a) contraindications exist.
   b) no contraindications exist.
8. Upon further examination of the ECG, you conclude that it shows:
   a) acute inferior STEMI.
   b) acute anterior STEMI.
   c) inferior myocardial infarction that may be old.
   d) anterior myocardial infarction that may be old.
   e) benign early repolarization changes.
   f) LBBB simulating anterior myocardial infarction.
   g) acute pericarditis.

   h) normal ECG.
   i) nonspecific ST changes.
 9. Your next procedural step should be to:
   a) order 0.4 mg sublingual nitroglycerin.
   b) order Maalox 30 cc po.
   c) order a gallbladder sonogram.
   d) order a repeat ECG in 15 min.

The patient reports no relief from sublingual nitroglycerin, and a repeat ECG is unchanged from the first.

10. At this point you conclude that:
   a) sufficient evidence of STEMI exists to initiate thrombolytic therapy.
   b) sufficient evidence of STEMI exists to initiate thrombolytic therapy if blood pressure can be reduced to below 180/110.
   c) evidence of STEMI exists, but absolute contraindications prohibit thrombolytic therapy.
   d) evidence of STEMI exists, but relative contraindications rule out thrombolytic therapy.
   e) insufficient evidence of STEMI exists to initiate thrombolytic therapy. Further workup is necessary to establish a diagnosis.
   f) insufficient evidence of STEMI exists to initiate thrombolytic therapy at present, but the index of suspicion is still high enough to warrant monitoring and repeat ECGs while a workup is proceeding.

Answers and Case Discussion

1. a   2. a   3. b   4. c   5. c   6. b   7. b   8. b   9. a   10. b

This middle-aged white female had significant risk factors in the form of obesity, hypertension, and diabetes, even though no family members were known to have had a myocardial infarction. Although the description of her pain, its radiation, and the way she related the pain to a fatty meal could suggest gallbladder disease, it is also entirely compatible with AMI. Nausea, vomiting, diaphoresis, and a mild sensation of shortness of breath could be common to both.

   Important aspects of the physical examination included wet skin and an S_4 gallop. Both findings are compatible with AMI, but wet skin can also be present in patients who are vomiting and in pain with acute cholecystitis, and an S_4 may be seen with hypertension alone. Nevertheless, the findings increase the index of suspicion for, and lend support to, a potential diagnosis of AMI.

   Measures taken immediately to protect life are always the most important, so starting an IV would be your first order of priorities as the physician responsible for this patient. As usual, a stat 12-lead ECG should be performed before a therapeutic trial of nitroglycerin.

   The ECG shows LAD with an axis of approximately −50 degrees, a small Q in lead I, and a small R wave in lead III. Criteria are present for LAH. ST-segment elevation is present in the anterior wall in V_1–V_3, with slight upwardly convex ST elevation also seen in leads I and aVL. Reciprocal depression is present in the inferior and lateral wall. Q waves have formed in leads V_1 and V_2, and there is only a tiny R wave left in V_3. These findings indicate acute anterior wall STEMI. A quick trial of nitroglycerin should be the next step to be certain that ST elevation is not on the basis of coronary artery spasm, although this is highly unlikely in the presence of developing Q waves.

Thrombolytic agents, on the basis of available information, are relatively contraindicated because of the patient's blood pressure in excess of 180/110, but should be administered if treatment is successful in reducing blood pressure to 180/110 or below. This can often be accomplished simply with morphine and nitroglycerin. Additional beta blockers should also be considered because she remains hypertensive with a heart rate in the 90s, despite being on oral metoprolol. Aspirin is not contraindicated because there is no reported allergy to aspirin.

Case 3

You are functioning as a staff nurse in the CCU of a rural community hospital on the night shift. Your hospital enjoys spectacular Smoky Mountain views, but the nearest tertiary medical center is 2.5 hours away by ground transport. It is 2:35 AM. One of your assigned patients is Mr. Fitzgerald, a 54-year-old white male auto parts dealer who was admitted to the CCU at 7:00 PM the evening before with a chief complaint of 20 min of retrosternal pressure that came on as he was walking to his car through the parking lot after closing. He reported that he had experienced similar discomfort three or four times in the last several weeks with walking long distances, but that previous episodes had never been this severe or lasted as long as 20 min.

His pain had faded by the time of arrival in the emergency department, and an initial ECG and enzyme studies had been negative. Nonetheless, he had been admitted to the CCU by his family physician with a preliminary diagnosis of unstable angina. Your review of the admitting nursing notes had revealed that he is a one and one-half pack a day smoker, and leads a sedentary lifestyle. He is on no medications, and actually has not seen a physician in several years. His father had coronary artery bypass surgery when he was 70 years of age. He has no known allergies.

Mr. Fitzgerald has a keep-vein-open IV line of 5% dextrose and water, and is connected to the ECG and noninvasive BP monitors. He is not on oxygen at present. His current medication orders include a nitroglycerin patch, metoprolol 50 mg po bid, Phenergan 12.5 mg IV q 2 h prn, Lovenox 70 mg sq q 12 h, and sublingual nitroglycerin 0.4 mg prn. You are sitting at the central monitoring station doing chart work when you hear his patient call bell.

As you enter the room you note that he remains in normal sinus rhythm and that his monitor is displaying a blood pressure of 108/86. As you grasp his hand and ask what he needs, you note that his skin feels cool and diaphoretic. Mr. Fitzgerald stoically reports that his retrosternal pain of earlier this evening returned approximately 30 min ago, but is now more severe. He appears uncomfortable and is moving almost constantly in the bed. Suddenly he sits up and emits a large amount of emesis.

1. Your first action would be to:
    a) administer 12.5 mg of Phenergan IV.
    b) start oxygen.
    c) administer 0.4 mg sublingual nitroglycerin.
    d) perform a 12-lead ECG.
2. Your second action would be to:
    a) administer 12.5 mg of Phenergan IV.
    b) start oxygen.
    c) administer 0.4 mg sublingual nitroglycerin.
    d) perform a 12-lead ECG.

Your quick preliminary physical exam reveals diaphoretic skin, no jugular venous distention, and clear lungs. Vital signs are a pulse of 78, respirations at 24, and BP of 108/86. A 12-lead ECG has been performed and is reproduced in Figure 14.3.

3. On the basis of currently available information, you conclude that thrombolytic agents, if necessary, would be:
    a) absolutely contraindicated.
    b) relatively contraindicated.
    c) not contraindicated.
4. With regard to contraindications to aspirin, should it be necessary, you conclude that:
    a) contraindications exist.
    b) no contraindications exist.
5. Upon completion of the ECG, you quickly note that the patient's electrocardiogram shows:
    a) a normal axis.
    b) RAD.

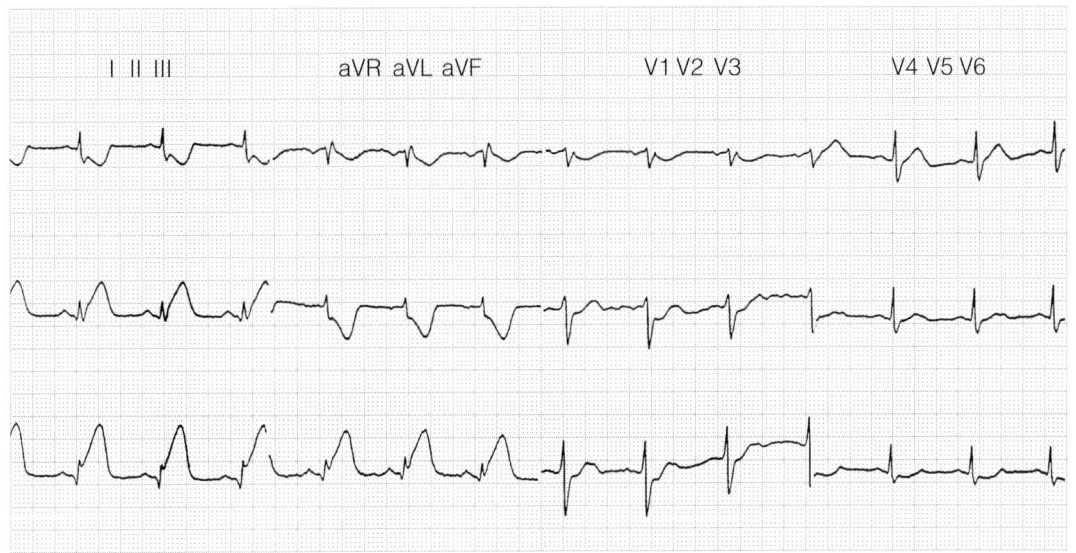

Figure 14.3.

    c) LAD.

    d) an indeterminate axis.

6. You place a call to the attending physician, report the events of the last 10 min, and report that it is your interpretation that the ECG shows:

    a) acute inferior STEMI.

    b) acute anterior STEMI.

    c) inferior myocardial infarction that may be old.

    d) anterior myocardial infarction that may be old.

    e) benign early repolarization changes.

    f) LBBB.

    g) RBBB.

    h) acute pericarditis.

    i) nonspecific ST changes.

    j) normal ECG.

7. When questioned by the physician, you further report that in your opinion:

    a) sufficient evidence of STEMI exists to recommend thrombolytic therapy.

    b) sufficient evidence of STEMI exists to recommend thrombolytic therapy if a therapeutic trial of sublingual nitroglycerin does not resolve ST-segment elevation.

    c) evidence of STEMI exists, but absolute contraindications prohibit thrombolytic therapy.

    d) evidence of STEMI exists, but relative contraindications rule out thrombolytic therapy.

    e) insufficient evidence of STEMI exists to recommend thrombolytic therapy.

Answers and Case Discussion

1. b   2. d   3. c   4. b   5. a   6. a   7. b

This middle-aged white male was admitted with an unsubstantiated clinical diagnosis of unstable angina. He carried risk factors of smoking and a sedentary lifestyle. His father clearly had coronary artery disease, although not at a terribly young age. The history of his chest discomfort over the preceding several weeks is a fairly typical one for new onset of angina.

    In the CCU, he develops recurrence of retrosternal pain associated with nausea, vomiting, and diaphoresis, certainly a symptom complex compatible with AMI. The diaphoresis present on physical exam increases our index of suspicion for AMI.

    The first appropriate step in this patient would be to start oxygen, an important step in protecting the patient that takes only seconds. The next step would be to immediately perform a 12-lead ECG. As discussed in previous cases, a therapeutic trial of nitroglycerin should be delayed until the ECG is performed to avoid obscuring the diagnosis.

    The ECG in this patient leaves little doubt as to the cause of his symptoms. The axis is normal at approximately 90 degrees, but there is dramatic ST elevation in leads II, III, and aVF, with reciprocal depression in leads I, aVL, and V_2–V_3. Early pathologic Q wave formation has also begun in leads III and aVF. It is a classic ECG of acute inferior wall STEMI.

There is nothing in the history to suggest contraindications to either thrombolytics or aspirin. The question arises as to whether or not to administer a therapeutic trial of nitroglycerin to someone who already has a nitroglycerin patch. In the absence of hypotension, most clinicians would still administer a dose of rapid acting nitroglycerin. Thrombolytic therapy is clearly indicated in this patient if a subsequent therapeutic trial of nitroglycerin does not resolve the ST elevation.

Case 4

Today you are again assigned to an ACLS unit in a large metropolitan area. It is 7:45 AM. Your unit is dispatched to an apartment building for chest pain and shortness of breath. In a fourth floor apartment you find 80-year-old Mr. Burgman wearing pajamas, sitting in his bedroom in a reclining chair. You immediately note that he appears very short of breath. Light from the bare overhead bulb is reflecting off his wet skin. As you approach his chair, you can hear respiratory wheezes even before you reach for your stethoscope. Multiple bottles of medication are scattered on the nightstand beside him. Mr. Burgman relates to you that he has been short of breath and his chest has felt very tight since approximately 5:00 AM. He is also nauseated, but has not yet vomited. He has broken out in a cold sweat in the last half hour.

With considerable effort, Mr. Burgman gasps that he has heart problems and has had three heart attacks, the last one a year ago. He has no known allergies. The medications on his nightstand include digoxin 0.125 mg qd, furosemide 40 mg bid, enalapril 5 mg bid, sublingual nitroglycerin 0.4 mg, and a box of transdermal nitroglycerin patches.

Your preliminary physical examination reveals an elderly white male who is in moderately severe respiratory distress and is able to speak in only short phrases because of dyspnea. Vital signs are a pulse of 92, respirations of 32, and a BP of 164/94. The skin is cool and damp. He is using his accessory muscles of inspiration. The neck veins are filled to the mandible. Basilar rales are present approximately a third of the way up the lung fields bilaterally, and there are diffuse expiratory wheezes. Heart sounds are distant, and they are obscured by the wheezes and rales. The underlying rhythm is regular, but you hear occasional premature beats. There is +1 peripheral pitting edema at the ankles.

1. With regard to the history, you conclude that:
   a) the history is adequate to be compatible with AMI.
   b) the history is incompatible with AMI.

While you have been gathering a brief history and performing your examination, your partner has placed Mr. Burgman on oxygen by nonrebreather mask, placed him on a cardiac monitor and pulse oximeter, and started an IV of NSS. The monitor shows him to be in normal sinus rhythm with occasional unifocal PVCs. His oxygen saturation is 88% on the nonrebreather mask.

2. Your next procedural step would be to:
   a) administer nitroglycerin 0.4 mg sublingually.
   b) administer furosemide 80 mg IV.
   c) perform a 12-lead ECG.
   d) administer lidocaine 75 mg IV.
   e) administer a unit dose of nebulized albuterol sulfate.
   f) start another twin-cath IV.
   g) administer 325 mg aspirin.
3. Your next procedural step would be to:
   a) administer nitroglycerin 0.4 mg sublingually.
   b) administer furosemide 80 mg IV.
   c) perform a 12-lead electrocardiogram.
   d) administer lidocaine 75 mg IV.
   e) administer a unit dose of nebulized albuterol sulfate.
   f) start another twin-cath IV.
   g) administer 325 mg aspirin.

While performing the above procedures, you are able to elicit no further history that would contraindicate thrombolytic therapy. An ECG has been performed and is now available to you as appears in Figure 14.4.

4. On the basis of currently available information, you conclude that thrombolytic agents, if they were to be needed, would be:
   a) absolutely contraindicated.
   b) relatively contraindicated.
   c) not contraindicated.
5. Upon completion of the ECG, you quickly note that the patient's electrocardiogram shows:

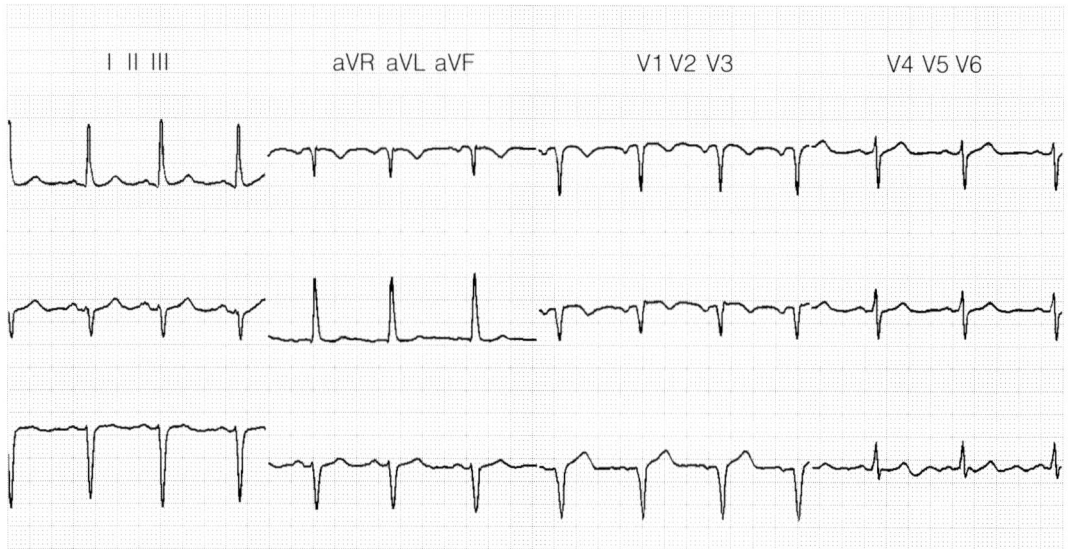

Figure 14.4.

a) a normal axis.

b) RAD.

c) LAD.

d) an indeterminate axis.

6. Upon further examination of the ECG you conclude that it shows

a) acute inferior STEMI

b) acute anterior STEMI

c) inferior myocardial infarction that may be old

d) anterior myocardial infarction that may be old

e) benign early repolarization changes

f) LBBB simulating anterior myocardial infarction

g) acute pericarditis

h) normal ECG

i) nonspecific ST changes

7. Your partner has established contact with medical command. Your field assessment as reported to the command physician is that:

a) sufficient evidence of STEMI exists to recommend thrombolytic therapy and to institute the prehospital thrombolytic protocol.

b) evidence of STEMI exists, but absolute contraindications prohibit thrombolytic therapy.

c) evidence of STEMI exists, but relative contraindications rule out thrombolytic therapy.

d) insufficient evidence of STEMI exists to recommend either thrombolytic therapy or implementation of the prehospital thrombolytic protocol.

e) insufficient evidence of STEMI exists to recommend thrombolytic therapy at present, but the index of suspicion is still high enough to warrant implementation of the prehospital thrombolytic protocol.

Answers and Case Discussion

1. a   2. b   3. c   4. c   5. c   6. d   7. e

Mr. Burgman is representative of a frequently encountered group of patients that can often be diagnostically challenging with regard to the presence or absence of AMI. He is an elderly patient with a long past medical history of cardiac disease, including his report of three previous heart attacks. His story of heart disease is corroborated by the medicines seen scattered on his nightstand. A quick glance at the patient as we enter the room is sufficient to tell us that he is in trouble. He is in acute respiratory distress and is diaphoretic. He reports tightness in his chest as well as shortness of breath.

Usually, at this early point we unconsciously begin to formulate a differential diagnosis in our minds and we begin to ask ourselves questions. When Mr. Burgman says his chest is tight does he mean that it is hard for him to take a breath because of the obvious bronchospasm, or does he mean that he has the constrictive feeling in his chest that people report with AMI? Is he short of breath and wheezing because he has chronic obstructive pulmonary disease with respiratory failure, or because he is in pulmonary edema?

A brief physical examination confirms that he is, indeed, in acute pulmonary edema. The presence of jugular venous distension, peripheral edema, rales at the bases, and his current array of medications that are aimed at congestive heart failure help us to feel confident that his respiratory distress is on the basis of pulmonary edema rather than chronic obstructive pulmonary disease with bronchospasm. Now we face the question of whether Mr. Burgman's problem is acute pulmonary edema alone, or whether it is acute pulmonary edema precipitated by AMI? Clearly the history is potentially compatible with both.

Before we have the luxury of answering that question, we must care for Mr. Burgman's immediately life-threatening problem. So our first procedural step would be to administer furosemide 80 mg IV, as we usually double the patient's oral dose when treating acute pulmonary edema. Nitroglycerin, of course, can also be beneficial in acute pulmonary edema by reducing preload and, to a lesser extent, afterload, but perhaps it would be best to wait until after an ECG has been performed to avoid the possibility of resolving ST-segment elevation before we have had the opportunity to see the ECG. Albuterol can also be useful as an adjunct for the reflex bronchospasm associated with pulmonary edema, but is not a first line drug for pulmonary edema. Mr. Burgman does have PVCs, but they are unifocal, and are seen only occasionally, so indications are not yet present for lidocaine.

With an IV established, and oxygen and furosemide now on board, we can perform a quick ECG. We have not yet discovered any contraindications to thrombolytic therapy, and we know that Mr. Burgman's age in and of itself is not a contraindication.

A glance at our ECG reveals that LAD is present with an axis of perhaps −40 or −50 degrees. A small R is present in lead III, and a small Q in lead I, so we are approaching criteria for LAH. We also note that the QRS duration approaches 0.10 s in some leads, so there appears to be a mild intraventricular conduction delay. Most striking, however, are the Q waves we see in V_1–V_3, indicating anterior wall infarction. The question then becomes is the infarction old or new? There is slight ST elevation of less than 2 mm in V_2 and V_3, but we know that slight ST elevation can often persist in the anterior wall after large anterior infarctions. If we look for reciprocal depression, there is none present on this tracing. We must conclude, therefore, that this tracing is most consistent with an old anterior myocardial infarction. Furthermore, we also know that Mr. Burgman reports that he has had a heart attack in the past, a history compatible with the finding of an old myocardial infarction on the ECG.

We are, thus, left with a history that is compatible with AMI, but not compelling for AMI. In addition, we have a history of previous myocardial infarction and an ECG that is more compatible with a remote infarction than with an acute infarction. Our assessment reported to med command should therefore be that there is insufficient evidence of STEMI to recommend thrombolytic therapy at the present, but because acute pulmonary edema is an occasional presenting symptom of AMI, prudence would dictate that we proceed with the prehospital protocol until subsequent evaluation in the emergency department (including a repeat ECG and most importantly, comparison to an old ECG) could enhance our confidence that STEMI was not present. Certainly we would not be surprised if a troponin performed in the emergency department came back positive, indicating a NSTEMI in this patient.

Although performing and assessing a field ECG takes only 3–4 min, additional measures to treat his pulmonary edema should take precedence over the ECG if this patient were to deteriorate or not improve after oxygen and furosemide. Such additional measures could include nitroglycerin, morphine sulfate, albuterol by nebulizer, or intubation.

Case 5

You are an independent primary health care provider working in a rural clinic in a western state. You are seventy 70 miles from the nearest hospital, so your clinic also functions as the region's only emergency facility. You therefore have access to all ACLS equipment and drugs, including thrombolytics. It is two o'clock in the afternoon.

Your receptionist has inserted a walk-in patient in your busy afternoon schedule because the patient is complaining of chest pain. You enter the room designated for emergencies and find a 54-year-old white female who appears anxious, but in no immediate distress. Your assistant has placed her on oxygen and has connected her to the cardiac monitor. You quickly note that the patient is in normal sinus rhythm.

Mrs. Anderson is a cook in your town's only restaurant. She is known county-wide for her chicken-fried steak. Her presence reminds you that you missed lunch and you are starving. You recall that you have been treating her with hydrochlorothiazide for mild hypertension for 3 years. She relates to you that she has had gradually increasing pain above her left breast and in her left shoulder and upper arm since approximately 10 AM today. She was unable to lift a frying pan with her left arm during the lunch rush today because of pain and weakness and had to use her right arm. There is no history of a previous similar pain. She denies nausea, vomiting, diaphoresis, or shortness of breath.

You glance at the patient chart and note the vital signs that have been recorded by your assistant: pulse 73, respirations 18, blood pressure 168/92. Mrs. Anderson is moderately obese. Her face is ruddy, but her skin is dry. There is no jugular venous distension. Her lungs are clear. Cardiac rhythm is regular without obvious gallops or murmurs. She is exquisitely tender to palpation over the head of her left biceps tendon. The abdomen is soft and nontender. There is no peripheral edema.

1. With regard to the pain, on the basis of currently available information you conclude that:
   a) the history is adequate to be compatible with AMI.
   b) the history is not compatible with AMI.
2. With regard to the physical examination, you conclude that:
   a) the physical exam lends support to the diagnosis of AMI.
   b) the physical exam neither confirms nor denies the possibility of AMI.
3. Your first procedural step would be to:
   a) start an IV of normal saline.
   b) administer nitroglycerin 0.4 mg sublingually.
   c) perform a 12-lead electrocardiogram.

A review of Mrs. Anderson's chart while the chosen procedure is being performed reveals only the past medical history of hypertension, and a hospitalization for a cystocele repair in 1984. Her parents are both still living. There is no history of bleeding, tumors, trauma, cerebrovascular accident, or recent surgery. She has no known allergies.

4. On the basis of currently available information, you conclude that thrombolytic agents, if they were to be needed, would be:
   a) absolutely contraindicated.
   b) relatively contraindicated.
   c) not contraindicated.
5. With regard to contraindications to aspirin, should it be necessary, you conclude that:
   a) contraindications exist.
   b) no contraindications exist.

An ECG has been performed and is now available to you. It is reproduced in Figure 14.5A.

6. Upon completion of the ECG, you quickly note that the patient's electrocardiogram shows:
   a) a normal axis.
   b) RAD.
   c) LAD.
   d) an indeterminate axis.
7. Upon further examination of the ECG, you conclude that it shows:
   a) acute inferior STEMI.
   b) acute anterior STEMI.
   c) inferior myocardial infarction that may be old.
   d) anterior myocardial infarction that may be old.
   e) benign early repolarization changes.
   f) LBBB simulating anterior myocardial infarction.
   g) RBBB.
   h) acute pericarditis.
   i) normal ECG.
   j) nonspecific ST changes.
8. Your next procedural step would be to:
   a) administer a therapeutic trial of nitroglycerin 0.4 mg sublingually.
   b) administer morphine sulfate 4 mg IV.
   c) compare the current ECG to an old one on the chart.

An ECG taken two years previously is shown in Figure 14.5B.

9. With regard to thrombolytic therapy, you conclude that:
   a) sufficient evidence of STEMI exists to initiate thrombolytic therapy and transport by helicopter to the nearest hospital.
   b) sufficient evidence of STEMI exists to initiate thrombolytic therapy if a therapeutic trial of sublingual nitroglycerin does not resolve ST segment elevation.
   c) evidence of STEMI exists, but absolute contraindications prohibit thrombolytic therapy.

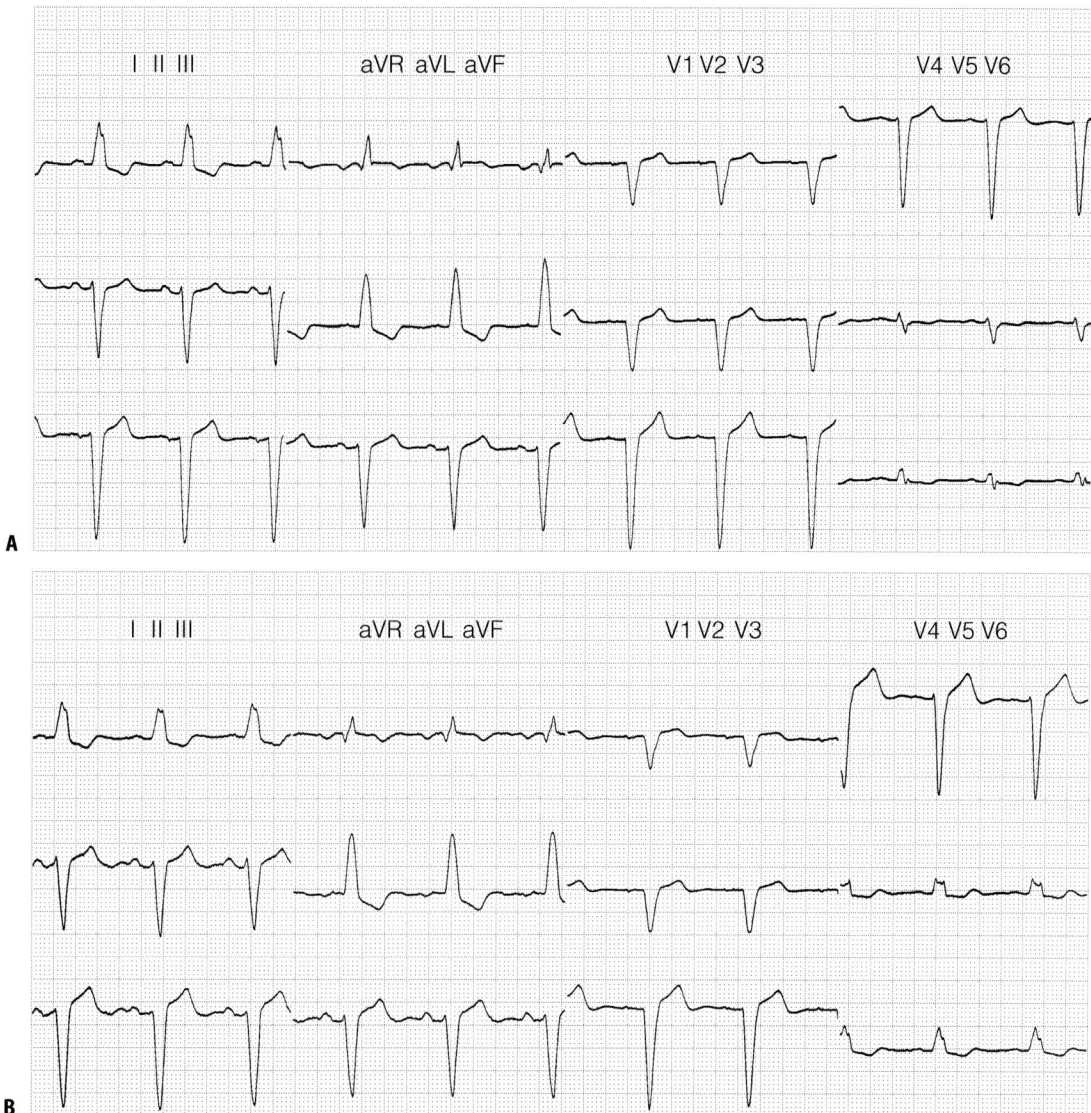

Figure 14.5.A.B.

d) evidence of STEMI exists, but relative contraindications rule out
   thrombolytic therapy.
e) insufficient evidence of STEMI exists to initiate thrombolytic therapy.

Answers and Case Discussion

1. b   2. b   3. c   4. c   5. b   6. c   7. f   8. c   9. e

Mrs. Anderson appeared in your clinic with a common presentation of chest
pain. Her pain was located in the upper left anterior chest, left shoulder, and

left upper arm. The most important historical finding is that the pain was clearly aggravated by the use of muscle groups in the same location as her pain. There is no history suggestive of unstable angina because she never had a previous similar pain. Nausea, vomiting, diaphoresis, and shortness of breath were absent. This is not a history compatible with AMI, but rather almost certainly represents chest wall pain coming from muscle inflammation or spasm.

The physical examination does nothing to heighten our index of suspicion for AMI, but rather supports a diagnosis of biceps tendonitis because she is exquisitely tender over the head of the biceps tendon. It is common for muscle or tendon inflammation in the left shoulder to radiate into the pectoral muscles of the left chest wall and vice versa. Nevertheless, we know that AMI frequently presents without cardiovascular abnormalities on physical examination, so for the sake of thoroughness, we prudently perform a 12-lead electrocardiogram. Because both the history and physical examination so clearly lend support to a diagnostic category of musculoskeletal pain, it is not necessary to start an IV at this time.

You may have been initially disquieted to see Mrs. Anderson's ECG. She has an intraventricular conduction delay because the QRS is 0.12 s or greater, and it is of the LBBB type. Her axis is approximately −70 degrees. We know that most bets are off with regard to diagnosing AMI in the presence of LBBB, so we are not very reassured by this electrocardiogram. We therefore look for an old ECG in her chart and find that she has had a LBBB for at least two years. We note that her current ECG is unchanged from the one on file. Now we can breathe easier. There is no evidence of AMI, and the history and physical examination are clearly compatible with biceps tendonitis. A week of rest and antiinflammatory medication and Mrs. Anderson will be back in the kitchen.

Case 6

You are a staff nurse in a lake resort community hospital emergency department. It is a busy summer Friday night at 9:30 PM and the place is packed. The sole physician on duty is suturing an extensive dog bite wound when the triage nurse brings back a 62-year-old black male with chest pain and hands the patient off to you. Mr. Frederick transfers from the wheelchair to the stretcher. He appears to be in pain. He relates to you that he has had retrosternal chest pain, radiating into both arms, for 30 min. As you are placing him on oxygen by nasal cannula at 6 L and connecting him to the monitoring equipment, you note that his skin appears warm and dry, and that he does not appear to be in respiratory distress. The monitor shows normal sinus rhythm at a rate of 80. The non-invasive blood pressure module reads 134/82. His oxygen saturation is 100% on oxygen. You quickly listen to his lungs, and they are clear. You can see no jugular venous distension. His heart rhythm is regular and you can hear no gross murmurs or gallops. His abdomen is soft and nontender. There is no peripheral edema.

You prepare to start an IV. Further questioning during this task reveals that he has been having chest discomfort about once a week for about two years. The discomfort usually comes with exercise, such as taking out the trash, and goes away within 2–3 min when he takes a nitroglycerin tablet or sits and rests for 5 min. He is maintained on diltiazem 60 mg tid and sustained release propranolol 80 mg bid. Tonight's pain came on at rest while watching TV after dinner, and it has been unrelieved by one sublingual nitroglycerin. He has never had pain this long. He has had no nausea and vomiting, diaphoresis, or shortness of breath. He denies allergies to medications.

1. With regard to the pain, on the basis of currently available information you conclude that:
   a) the history is adequate to be compatible with AMI.
   b) the history is not compatible with AMI.
2. With regard to the physical examination, you conclude that:
   a) the physical exam lends support to the diagnosis of AMI.
   b) the physical exam neither confirms nor denies the possibility of AMI.
3. You have completed starting the IV and have drawn bloods in the process. Your next step is to:
   a) administer 0.4 mg nitroglycerin sublingually.
   b) administer aspirin 325 mg PO.
   c) perform a STAT 12-lead electrocardiogram.
   d) start a second IV line.
   e) order a STAT portable chest film.

   Further questioning reveals no historical contraindications to thrombolytic therapy. A 12-lead ECG has been performed (Figure 14.6).

4. Upon completion of the ECG you quickly note that the patient's electrocardiogram shows:
   a) a normal axis.
   b) RAD.

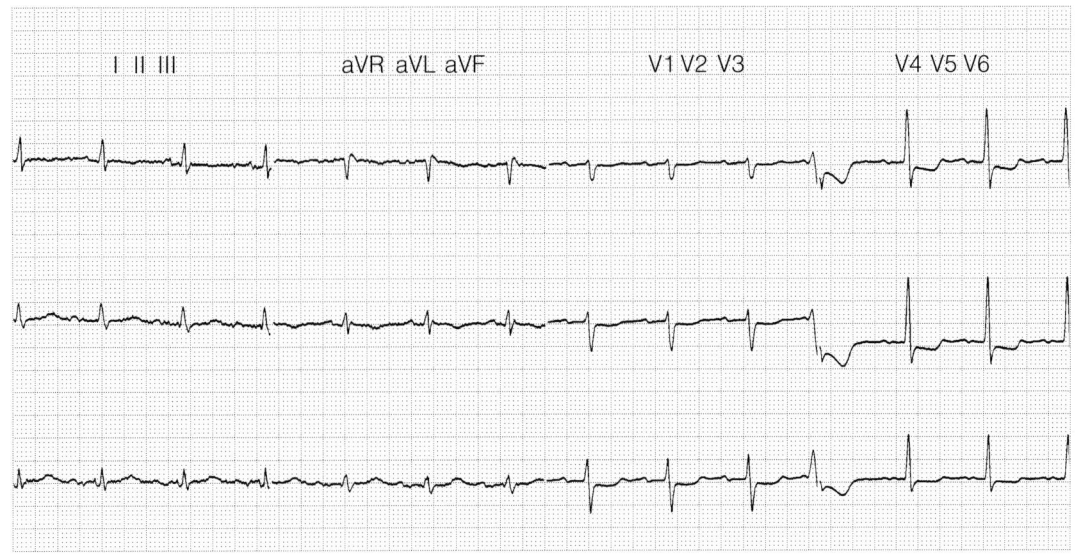

Figure 14.6.

    c) LAD.

    d) an indeterminate axis.

5. Upon further examination of the ECG you conclude that it shows:

    a) acute inferior STEMI.

    b) acute anterior STEMI.

    c) inferior myocardial infarction that may be old.

    d) anterior myocardial infarction that may be old.

    e) ST depression compatible with ischemia.

    f) LBBB simulating anterior myocardial infarction.

    g) RBBB.

    h) acute pericarditis.

    i) normal ECG.

    j) nonspecific ST changes.

6. After presenting a report to the physician, who is suturing the dog bite wound, and showing her the ECG, she is most likely to order you to:

    a) begin the thrombolytic protocol.

    b) start a nitroglycerin drip.

    c) complete the cardiac workup with a chest film.

    d) administer morphine sulfate 4 mg IV.

Answers and Case Discussion

1. a   2. b   3. c   4. a   5. e   6. b

This late middle-aged black male presents with a history of stable angina under current treatment with calcium channel blockers, beta blockers, and prn nitroglycerin. His pain usually comes with exertion, but today it came at rest and has continued for 30 min through to the time of admission. Although he has had no nausea, vomiting, diaphoresis, or shortness of breath, his pain almost certainly represents heart pain, and his symptoms are certainly compatible with AMI. We are not surprised that his physical examination is unrevealing, and we conclude that it neither confirms nor denies the possibility of AMI.

    We have taken measures to protect our patient from a sudden adverse event right up front with oxygen, monitoring, and starting an IV. Before we start any other form of therapy or do any other investigative test, our first order of business is now to obtain an ECG as quickly as possible. Up to this point, we have discovered no contraindications to thrombolytic therapy should the ECG reveal a STEMI.

    The ECG does not, however, show any ST elevation. Rather there is widespread ST depression of 2 mm or greater in leads V_4 and V_5. The ST segments are fairly straight and form a fairly acute angle with the T wave. This tracing is compatible with severe ischemia, but does not yet show AMI. At this point we have a classic case of unstable angina. In this context, our physician is most likely to order some form of nitroglycerin as the first and most important therapeutic step, now that the diagnosis seems confirmed. Other important diagnostic and therapeutic measures suited to acute coronary syndrome protocols will surely follow this first-line intervention.

Case 7

It is 11:30 AM on Sunday morning. Your ACLS unit is dispatched to a local church for chest pain. As you pull into the church parking lot a man is frantically waving toward the open church door. In the church vestibule a middle-aged white male is lying motionless, supine on the floor, his head in a pool of vomitus. A woman is kneeling over him, screaming hysterically. A teenager is giving the man closed chest massage, but he is not being ventilated. Your partner is already unpacking the defibrillator as you reach for a pulse, but none is present. As you rip open the man's shirt you ask a bystander how long ago he collapsed and he answers one minute, maybe two, before you arrived. The stricken man takes a sudden agonal gasp, but is otherwise not breathing.

1. Your first action will be to:
    a) start an IV.
    b) begin bag-valve-mask ventilation.
    c) connect to a monitor and defibrillate if ventricular fibrillation is present.
    d) intubate.

As the monitor baseline settles down you immediately recognize a pattern of coarse ventricular fibrillation. A shock at 200 joules is ineffective. After a second shock at 300 joules there is a brief moment of asystole, followed by return of a sinus bradycardia that slowly increases in rate to a sinus tachycardia. You are able to feel a brisk carotid pulse with each QRS.

2. You second action will be to:
    a) clear the airway and ventilate with bag-valve-mask while your partner assembles intubation gear.
    b) start an IV.
    c) administer epinephrine, 1 mg IV.
    d) administer lidocaine, 75 mg IV.

Your patient begins to breath spontaneously very shortly after defibrillation, and he is now beginning to stir. You decide not to intubate. As your partner starts the IV you learn from your patient's wife that he had 15 min of severe chest pain and broke out in a sweat before they got out of the pew and called 911. He vomited and then collapsed just before you arrived. His total period of arrest and CPR was probably under 4 min. His wife is not aware of any allergies. He is on no medications.

Lidocaine 75 mg IV, is now on board and a drip is running at 2 mg per minute. Mr. Seymour, as you now know his name to be, is moaning. His blood pressure is 132/78. His lungs are clear and he is moving air well. There is no suggestion of head trauma. He is being loaded onto the ambulance.

3. Your next action will be to:
    a) administer nitroglycerin spray under the tongue.
    b) perform a 12-lead ECG.

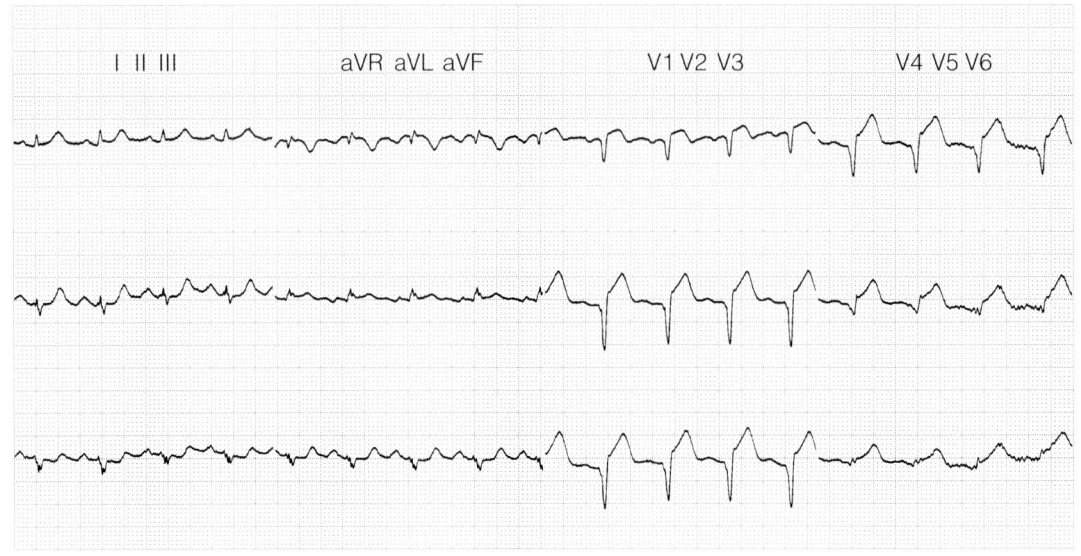

Figure 14.7.

c) administer aspirin 325 mg.
d) administer morphine sulfate 4 mg IV.

*A 12-lead ECG is now available to you and is pictured in Figure 14.7. Mr.
Seymour is now alert enough to answer most questions. You have discovered
nothing in his history that contraindicates thrombolytics.*

4. You quickly note that the patient's electrocardiogram shows:
    a) a normal axis.
    b) RAD.
    c) LAD.
    d) an indeterminate axis.
5. Upon further examination of the ECG, you conclude that it shows:
    a) acute inferior STEMI.
    b) acute anterior STEMI.
    c) inferior myocardial infarction that may be old.
    d) anterior myocardial infarction that may be old.
    e) ST depression compatible with ischemia.
    f) LBBB simulating anterior myocardial infarction.
    g) RBBB.
    h) acute pericarditis.
    i) normal ECG.
    j) nonspecific ST changes.
6. By this time you have concluded that thrombolytic therapy is:
    a) contraindicated.
    b) not contraindicated.
7. Radio contact has been established with medical command. Your field
    assessment, as reported to the command physician, is that:

a) sufficient evidence of STEMI exists to recommend thrombolytic therapy.

b) evidence of STEMI exists, but absolute contraindications prohibit thrombolytic therapy.

c) evidence of STEMI exists, but relative contraindications rule out thrombolytic therapy.

d) insufficient evidence of STEMI exists to recommend either thrombolytic therapy or implementation of the prehospital thrombolytic protocol.

e) insufficient evidence of STEMI exists to recommend thrombolytic therapy at present, but the index of suspicion is still high enough to warrant implementation of the prehospital thrombolytic protocol.

Answers and Case Discussion

1. c   2. a   3. b   4. c   5. b   6. b   7. a

Up to 40% of cases of AMI present to the Emergency Medical Services system as sudden death. This patient had a down time of only 1 or 2 min before ACLS arrival. Upon confirmation of absent pulse and respiration, the first priority is to rapidly establish what rhythm is present and administer DC countershock if the patient is determined to be in ventricular fibrillation.

The second priority in this case was to clear the airway, quickly ventilate with bag-valve-mask, and prepare to intubate. When patients have a short period of arrest and are rapidly defibrillated with return of good cardiac output, intubation is often not necessary if adequate spontaneous respirations quickly resume. Such was the case with this patient. Starting an IV and administering lidocaine are certainly appropriate measures in a patient who has just experienced ventricular fibrillation, but are secondary to adequate ventilation. Epinephrine was not indicated.

Mr. Seymour's history is a rather classic one for AMI complicated by early ventricular fibrillation. By now you are familiar with the concept that performance of the 12-lead ECG should be accomplished before administering nitroglycerin. Aspirin is not indicated until the decision has been made to institute the prehospital thrombolytic protocol, which requires the completion of a 12-lead ECG. Morphine is usually not administered until nitroglycerin has failed to provide pain relief.

Mr. Seymour's ECG shows an axis of −15 degrees, so LAD is present. Sinus tachycardia is present with a rate of slightly over 100. Prominent ST elevation is present in the anterior wall across the entire precordium, with reciprocal depression in the inferior wall indicating extensive anterior wall STEMI. Q waves have already formed in V_1–V_5.

There have been no contraindications to thrombolytic therapy elicited, and although CPR over 10 min is a relative contraindication, Mr. Seymour's period of resuscitation was no more than 4 min. Thrombolytic therapy is indicated in this patient, again, assuming that rapid PCI is not readily available in your region.

Case 8

It is 6:15PM. You are starving. You and your ACLS partner have just made your way through the cafeteria line and are sitting down to roast beef and lemon meringue pie when the tones go off. You are dispatched to a local residence for chest pain. Upon arrival, you recognize a familiar face. Mr. Saunders, who is 64-years-old, is well known to you, having a long history of coronary artery disease and having been transported to the hospital with chest pain three or four times in the last year and a half. His wife mentions to you that he was just discharged from the hospital two weeks ago after another heart attack.

Mr. Saunders reports to you that he is having retrosternal heaviness similar to that he has had in the past when he had heart attacks. You quickly note as you are placing him on oxygen that his skin is warm and dry, and that he does not appear dyspneic. As your partner connects him to the cardiac monitor, Mr. Saunders relates that he has had the pain approximately 15 min, but that he has no nausea, vomiting, or shortness of breath with the pain.

1. Your first action will be to:
   a) start an IV.
   b) administer sublingual nitroglycerin 0.4 mg.
   c) perform a 12-lead electrocardiogram.
2. Your second action will be to:
   a) start an IV.
   b) administer sublingual nitroglycerin 0.4 mg.
   c) perform a 12-lead electrocardiogram.

Questioning during the above procedures reveals that Mr. Saunders has had several heart attacks and several coronary stents placed in the past, and he was hospitalized for a bleeding ulcer about a year ago. He had at least one hospitalization for congestive heart failure. He is allergic to procainamide, but no other drugs. He is currently maintained on a nitroglycerin patch, furosemide 40 mg b.i.d., enalapril 10 mg b.i.d., Lanoxin 0.125 mg every other day, simvastatin 10 mg, and one aspirin daily. When asked specifically about "clot busting drugs" he thinks he was given one with his last heart attack two weeks ago, but is not sure what was the name of the drug.

Your brief physical examination has revealed a pulse of 96, respirations of 18, and a blood pressure of 108/68. Mr. Saunders has no jugular venous distention, his lungs are clear, you cannot hear a cardiac gallop (although there seems to be a systolic murmur present), and there is no peripheral edema.

3. By now you have concluded that thrombolytic therapy, should it be a therapeutic consideration, would be:
   a) contraindicated.
   b) relatively contraindicated.
   c) not contraindicated.

A 12-lead electrocardiogram has now been performed and is reproduced in Figure 14.8.

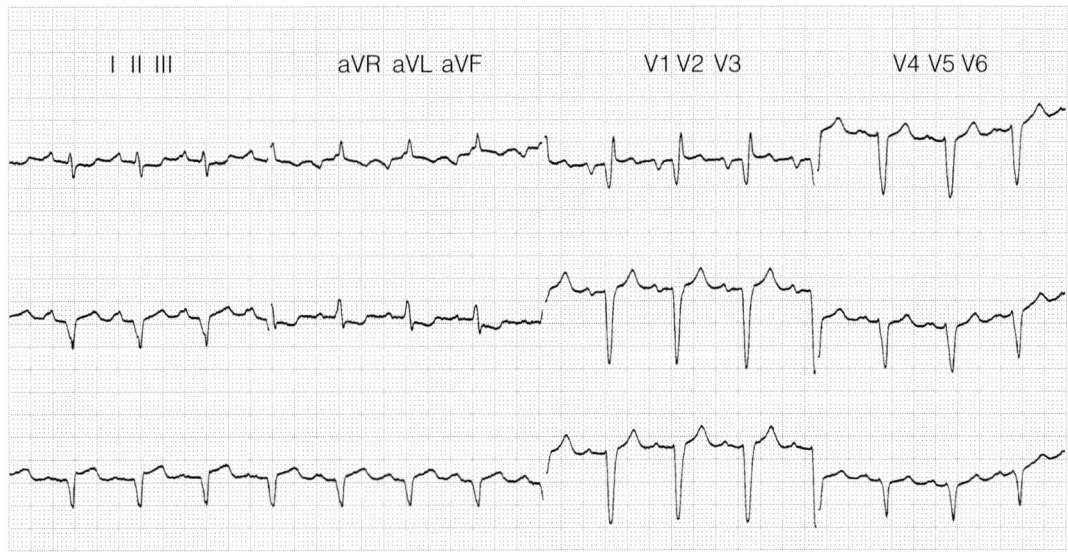

Figure 14.8.

4. You quickly note that the ECG shows an axis of approximately:
   a) −90 degrees.
   b) −60 degrees.
   c) 0 degrees.
   d) 60 degrees.
   e) 90 degrees.
5. Upon further examination of the ECG you conclude that it shows (you may select more than one answer):
   a) acute inferior STEMI.
   b) acute anterior STEMI.
   c) inferior myocardial infarction that may be old.
   d) anterior myocardial infarction that may be old.
   e) ST depression compatible with ischemia.
   f) LBBB simulating anterior myocardial infarction.
   g) RBBB.
   h) acute pericarditis.
   i) normal ECG.
   j) nonspecific ST changes.
6. Radio contact has been established with medical command. Your field assessment, as reported to the command physician, is that:
   a) sufficient evidence of STEMI exists to recommend thrombolytic therapy.
   c) evidence of STEMI exists, but absolute contraindications prohibit thrombolytic therapy.
   d) evidence of STEMI exists, but relative contraindications rule out thrombolytic therapy.
   e) insufficient evidence of STEMI exists to recommend either thrombolytic therapy or implementation of the prehospital thrombolytic protocol.

        f) insufficient evidence of STEMI exists to recommend thrombolytic therapy at present, but the index of suspicion is still high enough to warrant implementation of the prehospital thrombolytic protocol.

7. The medical command physician is now likely to recommend that you administer:

    a) aspirin, 325 mg chewed.
    b) nitroglycerin, 0.4 mg sublingually.
    c) morphine, 4 mg IV.
    d) lidocaine, 75 mg IV.

Answers and Case Discussion

1. a   2. c   3. c   4. a   5. a, d, g   6. f   7. b

Mr. Saunders is a very likely candidate for AMI. He has a history of several myocardial infarctions in the past, including one 2 weeks ago, as well as a history of congestive heart failure. His description of the pain that he is encountering this evening is that it feels about the same as the pain of his previous heart attacks. Clearly there is adequate history to have a very high index of suspicion for AMI.

You have a good partner who has already connected Mr. Saunders to the cardiac monitor while you were placing him on oxygen, and the last remaining immediate step to protect your patient would be to start an IV. Now you can perform a quick 12-lead ECG before nitroglycerin is administered.

By the end of your brief history and physical examination you should have concluded that thrombolytic therapy was not contraindicated. Mr. Saunders does have a history of a bleeding ulcer, but it was approximately a year ago, and does not contraindicate thrombolytic therapy. Indeed, he apparently had thrombolytic therapy with his last heart attack two months ago. Should you decide that thrombolytic therapy is indicated, you will need to check his old chart to see which thrombolytic agent was administered 2 months ago. If it was streptokinase, you would need to use another thrombolytic agent on this occasion because of the possible development of streptokinase antibodies.

Mr. Saunders' ECG shows extreme LAD. Lead aVR is upright, and lead I is equally biphasic, so we place the axis at approximately −90 degrees. Mr. Saunders' 12-lead ECG is very interesting and presents some real dilemmas. First, we note that the QRS duration is 0.12 s or greater, and that there is a very prominent R prime deflection in lead V_1. This means that Mr. Saunders has a RBBB. There is no R wave, however, in leads V_1 and V_2, and only the smallest of R waves in V_3 because Mr. Saunders has pathologic Q waves indicative of an anterior wall infarction. However, there is no acute anterior wall ST elevation, and no reciprocal depression in the inferior wall. Indeed, the inferior wall shows Q waves and ST elevation in leads II, III, and aVF. There is also some reciprocal depression in leads I and aVL, although there is none in the precordial leads. We therefore come to a tentative conclusion that the anterior wall infarction is probably old, but that the inferior wall infarction could be new because of the presence of inferior wall ST elevation and reciprocal depression in I and aVL.

Nevertheless, there is no reciprocal depression in V_1–V_3, and we also know that Mr. Saunders apparently just suffered a myocardial infarction two weeks ago. It is possible that the ST elevation in the inferior wall could be from a recent inferior wall infarction that has not yet undergone resolution. Thus, both the anterior and inferior infarctions could be old. In that case, his current chest pain could represent unstable angina. Clearly, we are going to need to see an old tracing from his recent hospitalization before we can confidently tell whether the inferior wall infarction is new, or was suffered two weeks ago.

Because both the anterior and inferior wall infarctions may be old, we can not currently recommend institution of thrombolytic therapy, but can only recommend that the index of suspicion is still high enough to warrant proceeding to implement the prehospital thrombolytic protocol. Final decisions will have to await comparison of our field ECG with Mr. Saunders' old ECG in the emergency department.

Because Mr. Saunders is already taking an aspirin daily, our medical commander is likely to order sublingual nitroglycerin, now that we have obtained a 12-lead ECG.

So what was the outcome of this case? It was unstable angina. Mr. Saunders' field ECG, upon comparison to old tracings in the emergency department, was essentially unchanged from his last tracing 2 weeks before when he was discharged following an acute inferior wall myocardial infarction. Very challenging case. If you got all seven questions right in this case, you get a star.

Case 9

Despite the pressures of too many patients being jammed into every day's schedule, commuting 20 min each way to the hospital, and the necessity of taking call every other night, rural family practice has always been your first love. This evening is no exception with a waiting room full of coughing kids, pregnant young mothers, and the usual assortment of diabetics and hypertensives. You enter Exam Room 3 to see Ray Stoneham, a cheerful 68-year-old dairy farmer with a ruddy complexion and a concerned wife who talked your receptionist into sticking him into tonight's packed schedule.

His wife preempts your attempt to take a history by announcing that Ray has had indigestion for three days, has been taking Tums by the bucketload, and just picks at his food. She is sure that he has an ulcer.

Ray seems content with his wife running this show, and makes no effort to offer further clarification. The office chart in your hand is thin. Ray normally comes in only when coerced by his wife. He has never been in a hospital, has no chronic illnesses, no allergies, and is on no meds. But tonight, his wife says, he himself suggested going to the doctor's office. Gradually you are able to coax more information out of Ray and you learn that his indigestion is high in the retrosternal area, has been constant for almost three days, and seems worse when he is carrying feed to the calves. In fact, he felt badly enough that he did not milk the cows tonight, but left that task to his son-in-law. He vomited once the first night of the indigestion and was sweaty most of the night. Tums have not seemed to relieve the indigestion.

During your questioning you are working your way through a brief physical examination. You note that Ray's skin is warm and dry. There is no jugular venous distension. His lungs are clear. His cardiac rhythm is regular, in the 80s with an occasional premature beat. There are no murmurs or gallops. His abdomen is soft and nontender. You are unable to reproduce his discomfort with palpation in the epigastrium. You note on the chart that his blood pressure is 148/92.

1. Your next step would be to:
   a) call an ambulance.
   b) schedule an upper GI series.
   c) schedule a gall bladder sonogram.
   d) perform a stat electrocardiogram.
   e) order screening chemistries and enzymes.
   f) start O_2, an IV, and connect to your office monitor/defibrillator.
2. Your second step would be to:
   a) call an ambulance.
   b) schedule an upper GI series.
   c) schedule a gall bladder sonogram.
   d) perform a stat electrocardiogram.
   e) order screening chemistries and enzymes.
   f) start O_2, an IV line, and connect Ray to your office monitor/ defibrillator.

An ECG has been performed and is now available (see Figure 14.9). There is no old tracing on file for comparison.

3. By now you have concluded that thrombolytic therapy, should it be a therapeutic consideration, would be:

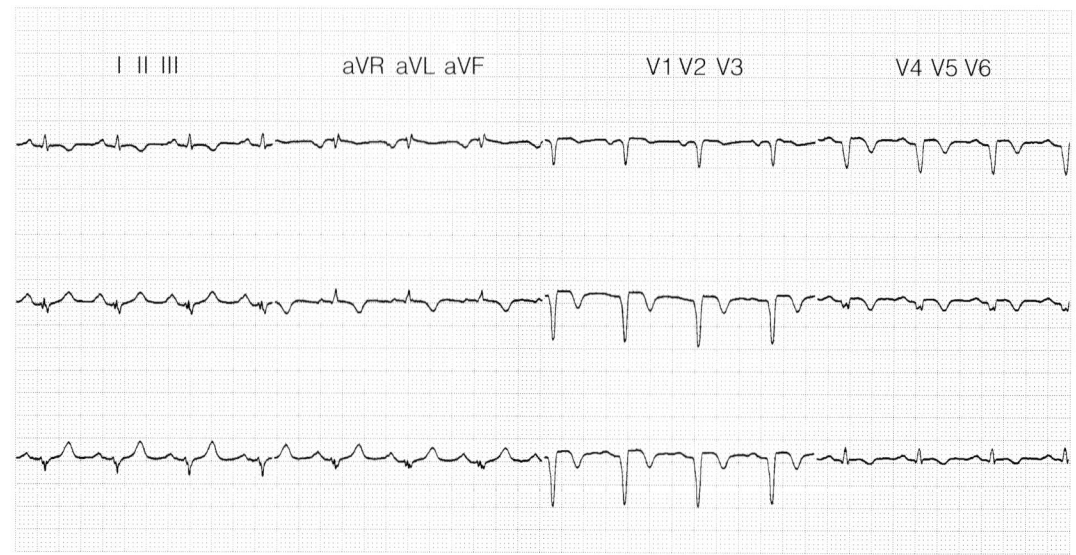

Figure 14.9.

    a) contraindicated.
    b) relatively contraindicated.
    c) not contraindicated.
4. You quickly note that Mr. Stoneham's tracing shows:
    a) LAH.
    b) LPH.
    c) nonspecific intraventricular conduction delay.
    d) RBBB.
    e) LBBB.
    f) normal QRS duration and axis.
5. In addition, Mr. Stoneham's tracing shows:
    a) evolving acute inferior STEMI.
    b) evolving acute anterior STEMI.
    c) inferior myocardial infarction that may be old.
    d) anterior myocardial infarction that may be old.
    e) ST depression compatible with ischemia.
    f) LBBB simulating anterior myocardial infarction.
    g) RBBB.
    h) acute pericarditis.
    i) normal ECG.
    j) nonspecific ST changes.
6. By this time you have concluded that Mr. Stoneham:
    a) is a candidate for thrombolytic therapy.
    b) is not a candidate for thrombolytic therapy.
7. Your next step would be to:
    a) call an ambulance.
    b) schedule an upper GI series.
    c) schedule a gall bladder sonogram.
    d) order screening chemistries and enzymes.
    e) start O_2, an IV, and connect to your office monitor/fibrillator.

Answers and Case Discussion

1. f   2. d   3. c   4. a   5. b   6. b   7. a

Ray Stoneham is typical of a group of stoic patients who endure symptoms of cardiac disease and convince themselves that their symptoms represent something less serious. The first hint that this is not a GI problem comes when Ray relates that his "indigestion" is in the high retrosternal area. Aggravation of the pain with exercise sets off further alarm bells. Vomiting and diaphoresis the first night of the pain complete the transition to a focus on a possible cardiac etiology. Ray's symptoms, indeed, are sufficiently worrisome to warrant hospitalization regardless of our findings on physical examination or laboratory investigation.

    The physical exam is not particularly helpful. The only positive finding is that there is an occasional premature beat, which, in and of itself, does not significantly heighten our index of suspicion for AMI. The absence of tenderness in the epigastrium does help to heighten our suspicion that this illness is not gastrointestinal in etiology.

On the basis of the history alone, which is highly suspicious for AMI, our initial step would be to start O2, connect to a monitor/defibrillator, and start an IV, if all were available in the office, to protect Ray from an adverse event like ventricular fibrillation. Our next step would be to perform a stat electrocardiogram.

There is nothing in Ray's history that suggests a contraindication to thrombolytics, although you may have chosen "a) contraindicated" to question number 3 because he has had the pain for three days; outside the window for thrombolytic therapy. If so, go ahead and give youself credit.

Ray's electrocardiogram is illuminating. LAD of approximately –45 degrees, and a small Q in lead I and a small R in lead III meet criteria for LAH. Most disturbing, however, are the Q waves in V_1–V_3 with deep T wave inversion characteristic of an anterior wall STEMI in evolution. The question of how old this infarction is arises. T wave inversion takes hours to days to evolve, at least, so the ECG would suggest that it is probably at least more than several hours old.

Often, however, the most accurate way to judge the age of an evolving infarction is on the basis of the patient's history. Ray tells us that his pain has been constant for nearly 3 days, and that on the first night of the pain he had diaphoresis and vomiting. Clinically, then, the infarction commenced 3 days ago. Too late for thrombolytic therapy, but still early enough that he remains at some risk and should be hospitalized. Other interventions should now be taken, probably including nitrates and beta blockers, as well as antiplatelet therapy, and perhaps anticoagulation. His continuing pain, suggesting ongoing ischemia, may lead a consulting cardiologist to refer him for urgent PCI. Our final step in question 6, then, would be to call 911 for an ambulance trip to the hospital with ACLS services.

Case 10

When Robert Freuf was   admitted to the coronary care unit, you learned during your nursing evaluati   ion that Robert was unfortunate enough to have had a myocardial infarcti... even years previously at the age of 33. Robert had a cardiac catheterization shortly thereafter, the results of which are unclear to you. He can only remember that they told him he had a "tear" in a vessel wall. After 7 years free of chest pain, or other symptoms, Robert had been readmitted 2 weeks ago with a several week history of exertional chest discomfort relieved by rest, and then, finally, an episode of pain at rest, leading to admission. After several days in the CCU, Robert had had a treadmill stress test performed, which was negative, and he was discharged on aspirin and simvastatin.

Late this afternoon, Robert again experienced an hour of severe retrosternal chest discomfort that began to ease at about the time of admission to the emergency department. Robert's emergency department ECG at 5:37 PM is seen in Figure 14.10. It is unchanged from that of his previous admission. He reported to the emergency department staff that he had taken his aspirin and simvastatin that morning.

1. Robert's emergency department ECG at 5:37 PM shows:
   a) LAH.
   b) LPH.

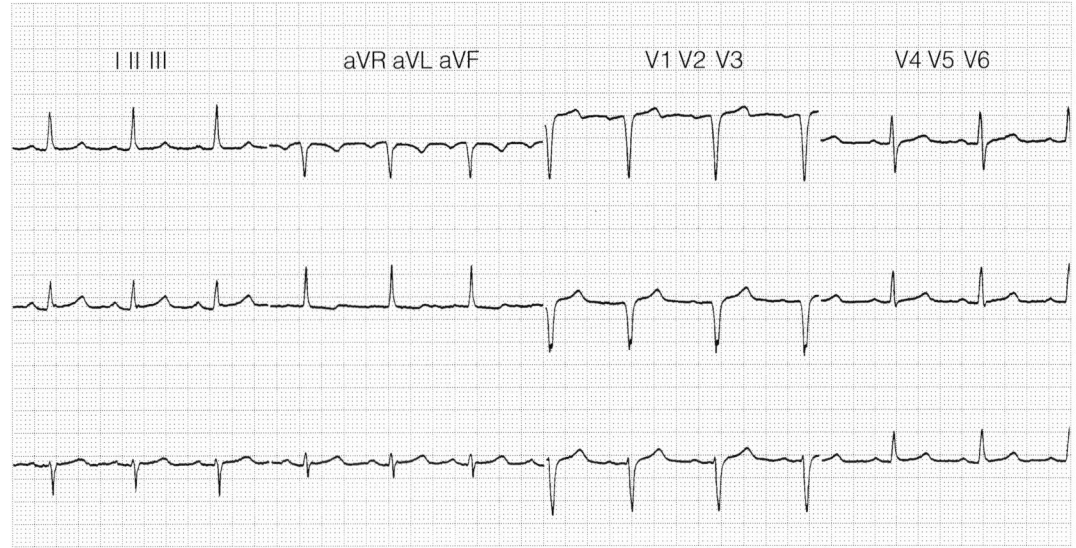

Figure 14.10.

    c) nonspecific intraventricular conduction delay.
    d) RBBB.
    e) LBBB.
    f) normal QRS duration and axis.
2. In addition, Robert's 5:37 PM tracing shows:
    a) acute inferior STEMI.
    b) acute anterior STEMI.
    c) inferior myocardial infarction that may be old.
    d) anterior myocardial infarction that may be old.
    e) ST depression compatible with ischemia.
    f) LBBB simulating anterior myocardial infarction.
    g) RBBB.
    h) acute pericarditis.
    i) normal morphology.
    j) nonspecific ST changes.

Robert has been pain-free since admission to the CCU 45 min ago. He is on oxygen at 2 liters by nasal cannula, has a keep-vein-open IV of 5% dextrose and water, and has a nitroglycerin drip running at 26 mic/min. He received 50 mg of atenolol by mouth at 6:15 PM. His physician has written prn orders for morphine and an antacid. At approximately 6:30 PM he rings his call bell and when you enter the room tells you that the pain has returned. He rates the pain as an 8 on a scale of 10.

3. Your first step would be to:
    a) increase the rate of the nitroglycerin drip.
    b) take vital signs and do a brief pertinent physical examination.
    c) administer morphine sulfate 4 mg IV.
    d) perform a repeat 12-lead electrocardiogram.
    e) administer Maalox 30 ml PO.

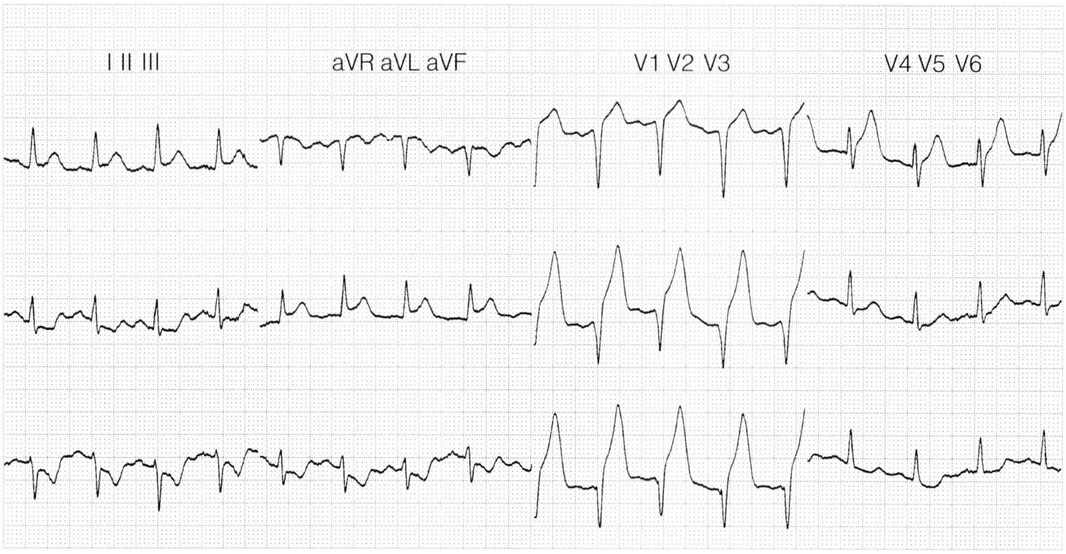

Figure 14.11.

4. Your second step would be to:
   a) increase the rate of the nitroglycerin drip.
   b) take vital signs and do a brief pertinent physical examination.
   c) administer morphine sulfate 4 mg IV.
   d) perform a repeat 12-lead electrocardiogram.
   e) administer Maalox 30 ml PO.

   Robert's current vital signs are a pulse of 103, BP of 158/92, and respirations of 20. His skin is cool and slightly diaphoretic. There is no jugular venous distension. His lungs are clear and there is no suggestion of a new murmur or gallop rhythm. A 12-lead electrocardiogram taken at 6:38 PM is reproduced in Figure 14.11.

5. Robert's 6:38 PM tracing shows:
   a) acute inferior STEMI.
   b) acute anterior STEMI.
   c) inferior myocardial infarction that may be old.
   d) anterior myocardial infarction that may be old.
   e) ST depression compatible with ischemia.
   f) LBBB simulating anterior myocardial infarction.
   g) RBBB.
   h) acute pericarditis.
   i) normal morphology.
   j) nonspecific ST changes.
6. Your next step would be to:
   a) increase the rate of the nitroglycerin drip.
   b) take vital signs and do a brief pertinent physical examination.
   c) administer morphine sulfate, 4 mg IV.
   d) question patient regarding thrombolytic contraindications and prepare for possible thrombolytic therapy.
   e) administer Maalox 30 ml PO.
   f) administer aspirin 325 mg PO.

Robert has received no relief of pain from the measures taken so far. You have been unable to contact Robert's physician by either pager or telephone. You have left him connected to the 12-lead ECG machine, and you note that there is no change from the previous 6:38 PM tracing.

7. Your next step would be to:
   a) increase the rate of the nitroglycerin drip.
   b) take vital signs and do a brief pertinent physical examination.
   c) administer morphine sulfate, 4 mg IV.
   d) question patient regarding thrombolytic contraindications and prepare for possible thrombolytic therapy.
   e) administer Maalox, 30 ml PO.
   f) administer aspirin, 325 mg PO.

Answers and Case Discussion

1. f   2. d   3. b   4. d   5. b   6. a   7. d

This case illustrates the importance of maintaining a high index of suspicion and performing repeat ECGs in patients whose symptoms change. Robert is young and had a recent admission with a negative workup. In addition, although his emergency department ECG shows LAH and Q waves consistent with an old anterior myocardial infarction, it is unchanged from that of his previous admission. It is easy to be lulled into a false sense of security by this history of a negative workup and continued negative ECGs without acute changes.

But once again, 45 min after admission, Robert experiences a return of his chest pain. As always, when a patient's condition changes, we need to check the patient. So the first step would be taking his vital signs and, at the very least, observing skin color and temperature, checking for jugular venous distension, and listening to his heart and lungs.

It would be tempting at this point to increase the nitroglycerin drip in an effort to relieve Robert's pain, but as we have learned in earlier cases, it is better to quickly perform a 12-lead ECG first to not miss a diagnosis.

The 12-lead ECG performed at 6:38 leaves no doubt as to the etiology of Robert's pain. Dramatic ST elevation is present in the anterior wall with reciprocal depression. It is now time to turn up the nitroglycerin drip to see if higher doses relieve the pain and ST elevation.

You have prudently left Robert connected to the 12-lead machine (or, if you have ST-segment monitoring in your CCU, you may have continuously monitored his ST segments). In the absence of relief, it is time to begin questioning the patient with regard to contraindications to thrombolytic therapy and prepare for thrombolytic therapy in anticipation of it being ordered, assuming unavailability of immediate PCI.

You may be interested to hear that in the real-life case, Robert's ST-segment elevation and pain resolved within approximately 10 min of increasing the nitroglycerin drip. He was started on a heparin drip and flown to a tertiary center where he underwent emergency cardiac catheterization, which revealed three-vessel obstructive coronary artery disease not very amenable to stenting. Immediately thereafter he was taken to the operating room where he underwent an uncomplicated triple coronary artery bypass.

Case 11

When 59-year-old Clifford Bumbaugh walked up to the receptionist's counter in your ER, even the receptionist knew immediately that Clifford, the hospital's night shift maintenance man, was in trouble. He was pale as a ghost, sweat dripped off his nose onto the registration log, and he leaned on the counter with one hand, and clutched his chest with the other.

But all your hard work in training the staff of your little rural community hospital rapidly pays off. Clifford is whisked away in a wheelchair by the triage nurse, and within five min, his primary nurse has tracked you down and presented you with the ECG in Figure 14.12. As she hands you the ECG, she announces that Clifford has had pain for only 20 min and has no contraindications to fibrinolytics. By the time you reach the room, another team nurse informs you that Clifford has received four baby aspirin and has had a spray of nitroglycerin under his tongue. Six minutes have now elapsed since door-time. You give a little smile of self-satisfaction at the performance of your staff.

Two nurses are starting IVs, one in each arm, as you approach the bed. You glance at the monitor and note a heart rate of 59 and a blood pressure of 90/52.

1. Clifford's ECG at 10:37 PM reveals:
   a) LVH with a strain pattern.
   b) evidence of RVH.
   c) a normal axis and QRS duration.
   d) an intraventricular conduction delay.
   e) RBBB.
2. In addition, Clifford's 10:37 PM tracing shows:
   a) evidence of anterior wall ischemia compatible with unstable angina.
   b) an anteroseptal STEMI.
   c) nonspecific ST and T wave changes.
   d) an inferior wall STEMI.
   e) acute pericarditis.
   f) an anterior wall NSTEMI.

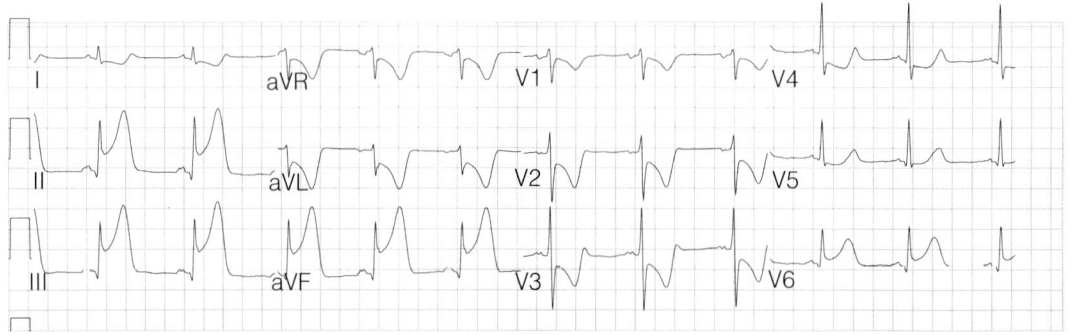

Figure 14.12.

3. Your first action should be to:
   a) question Clifford about the nature of his pain.
   b) feel each radial and femoral pulse while questioning him.
   c) order a second ECG to check for resolution of ST segment elevation.
   d) do all of the above at the same time.

Cliff tells you that the pain is like someone is blowing up a balloon inside him and, despite the pain on his face, makes a weak joke about having your penknife on you to prick the balloon. He denies radiation from the retrosternal region. He has never had a pain like this before. There is no history of hypertension. Pulses seem equal to your fingertips, bilaterally. You quickly do a mini–cardiovascular exam. Clifford's neck veins aren't up, his lungs are clear, he has no gallops or murmurs, and you can feel no pulsatile masses in his belly. While palpating his belly, you ask all the bleeding questions and he replies in the negative. A second ECG looks just like the first. Cliff is still in a lot of pain and asks for his wife. Eight minutes have now elapsed from door-time.

4. At this point you:
   a) order a nitroglycerin drip starting at 13 mics.
   b) order metoprolol 5 mg IV every 5 min for three doses.
   c) have the ward clerk get the 24-hour cath lab at a tertiary center 30 min away by helicopter on the line and order a helicopter for transport for emergent PCI.
   d) obtain informed consent from Clifford and order thrombolytics.
   e) order a portable chest film.
5. The next order of business is to order:
   a) a nitroglycerin drip starting at 13 mics.
   b) metoprolol 5 mg IV every 5 min for 3 doses.
   c) morphine sulfate 4 mg IV.
   d) a CT of the chest.

Twenty minutes after your chosen action in question number three above, Clifford is noted to have ST-segment elevation in lead aVF of approximately 2.5 mm. His pain is now down from a "10" to a "2" and his skin is drying.

6. You conclude that:
   a) the nitroglycerin drip is producing some relief of his ischemia.
   b) Clifford is now developing an acute inferior wall STEMI.
   c) evidence is accumulating of possible reperfusion.
   d) the time has come for immediate transfer for emergent PCI.

Things are going pretty well. Cliff's BP is now 98/68 and his heart rate is in the low 60s. His wife is seated on a folding chair at his bedside, holding Cliff's hand. Seventeen-year-old Cathy Bumbaugh, the apple of her father's eye, lounges against the railing on the other side of the bed. Cliff is talking about bass fishing when his sentence trails off into a low moan, his head rolling to one side. Pandemonium breaks out. Mrs. Bumbaugh gasps and jumps to her feet, the chair clattering to the floor behind her. From the central station across

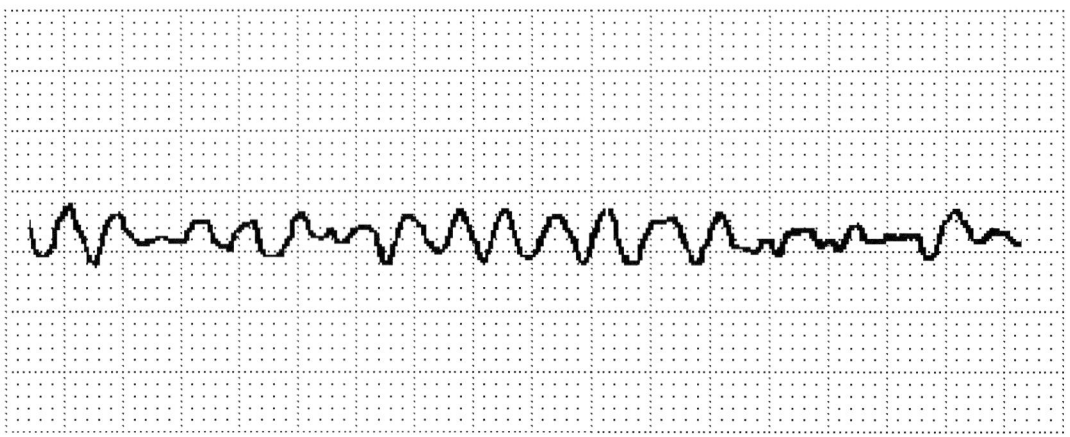

Figure 14.13.

the hall you hear Cathy scream, "Daddy?" At the same time an alarm begins to clang and you glance toward the central monitoring bank. You see the rhythm strip in Figure 14.13 go across the screen.

7. The appropriate first intervention would be to:
    a) rapidly intubate.
    b) shock at 200 J.
    c) administer 300 mg amiodarone IV.
    d) administer 100 mg lidocaine IV.

After Cliff regains consciousness he begins to moan and complain of chest pain again. He has received a bolus of 100 mg of lidocaine and a drip has been started. It is now 35 min from "needle time." You run another 12-lead ECG and it looks almost identical to Figure 14.12.

8. Your next priority would be to:
    a) administer another 4 mg morphine sulfate IV.
    b) increase the nitroglycerin drip to 26 mics.
    c) have the ward clerk get the 24-hour cath lab at a tertiary center 30 min away by helicopter on the line and order a helicopter for transport for emergent rescue PCI.
    d) Start an amiodarone drip.

Answers and Case Discussion

1. c   2. d   3. d   4. d   5. c   6. c   7. b   8. c

Clifford's case happened in real life, and I'll tell you the outcome shortly. The real case was filled with the same ambiguities and tough decisions you faced in trying to decide proper management while reading the case. I hope everyone got the first and second answers correct; Cliff had a normal axis and QRS duration, but dramatic evidence of acute inferior wall ST segment elevation infarction, including tall, peaked hyperacute T waves.

Question 3, of course, was aimed at reinforcing the concept that in the provider-patient encounter you can accomplish many things rapidly at the same time, and was aimed particularly at reinforcing the concept that you need to always keep the possibility of aortic dissection at the front of your mind when faced with a clinical STEMI and the potential for fibrinolysis.

The next narrative paragraph sets the stage for the most complex decision-making of the case and brings to the forefront some controversial issues. These issues include when patients with STEMI in community hospitals should be transferred to tertiary institutions for primary PCI, how far one should go in ruling out aortic dissection before committing to fibrinolytics, and subjective decisions regarding the priority of beta blockers and nitroglycerin in patients with hypotension and slow heart rates. I will tell you now that a group of a dozen cardiologists would not all agree on the answers to some of the difficult questions that were faced with Cliff.

Cliff presented early, after only 20 min of pain. It took only 6 min from door time to make the diagnosis of STEMI. If a helicopter was ordered at that time it would take "scramble time" (perhaps 3 min) plus a 30 minute flight time to arrive at your facility. Another 10 min for loading, a return trip of 30 min to the tertiary center, and 10 min to prep and gain catheter access would total approximately 80 min. If everything went perfectly smoothly, Cliff could perhaps have PCI accomplished in under the 90-minute period allotted to accomplish primary PCI in the ACC Guidelines.

However, with the opportunity to make a thrombolysis decision occurring at only 8 min after arrival, the staff was able to achieve a door to needle time of only 10 or 12 min. Thus, choosing primary PCI would have created a time difference of approximately 70 min between opportunity for thrombolysis and opportunity for primary PCI, exceeding the 60 min advocated by the ACC Guidelines as being the maximum recommended time difference between thrombolysis and PCI. Cliff therefore received TNK in real life.

You will note that the decision to thrombolyse was made without benefit of a chest film. A chest X-ray, although useful if immediately available, is not required to rule out a dissection. Cliff did not relate the tearing kind of pain usually associated with dissection, it did not radiate to his back, and he had equal pulses bilaterally. Most authorities agree that this constitutes adequate clinical clearance for thrombolysis. Indeed, in the realm of prehospital thrombolysis, there is no radiologic imaging option. As is usually the case in medicine, you're playing the odds.

As is often typical with inferior STEMIs, Cliff had a heart rate in the high 50s and a BP of approximately 90. Nitrates and beta blockers would likely push Cliff's blood pressure down to undesirable levels, and his heart rate was already at levels usually achieved with beta blockers, so pain control was given the priority in question 5. Note that the morphine was given in a relatively small dose to try to avoid further hypotension. Also remember that when choosing between nitrates and beta blockers in acute coronary syndromes, greater value accrues to the beta blocker, and it should always be given priority over nitrates in patients with marginal blood pressures.

The next narrative paragraph tells us that Cliff's ST segments have come down 2.5 mm, or approximately 50% from their high of 5 mm in his initial

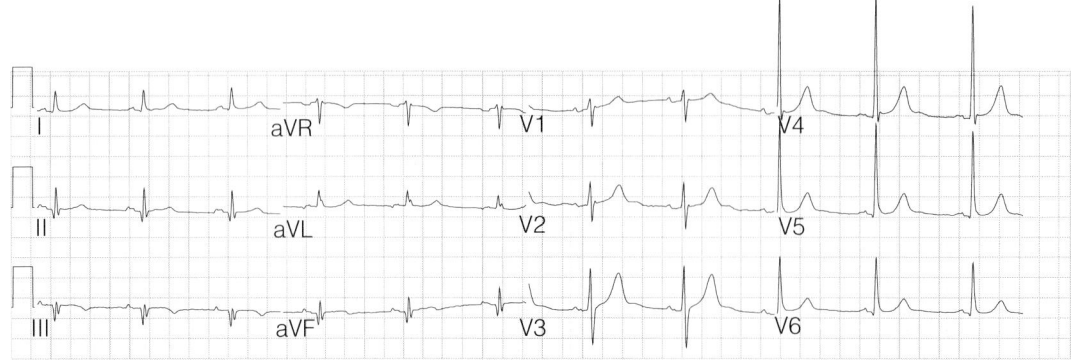

Figure 14.14.

ECG. In addition, his pain is much better. This constitutes provisional evidence of reperfusion.

Unfortunately, an episode of ventricular fibrillation ensues, and after a successful defibrillation, Cliff develops more pain and his ST segments return to nearly 5 mm. We must now conclude that Cliff has suffered a reocclusion despite thrombolysis. It is now time to move rapidly and aggressively to facilitate transport to a cath lab for rescue PCI.

That's exactly what happened to the real-life Cliff. Cliff had a 95% proximal RCA occlusion at the time of PCI. Happily enough, his post-PCI ECG in Figure 14.14 reflects resolution of ST changes, although Q waves are present in the inferior wall that suggest Cliff may still have lost some muscle.

Answers to Practice Tracings

Chapter 5

Figure 5.5: −5 degrees.
Figure 5.6: Slightly >90 degrees.
Figure 5.7: 140 degrees.
Figure 5.8: −20 degrees.

Chapter 6

Figure 6.8: LPH; axis 115 degrees.
Figure 6.9: LAH; axis −45 degrees.
Figure 6.10: LPH; axis 175 degrees.
Figure 6.11: LAH; axis −70 degrees.

Chapter 7

Figure 7.19: Complete LBBB; axis −20 degrees.
Figure 7.20: Incomplete LBBB; axis −7 degrees.
Figure 7.21: Complete RBBB and LAH; axis −55 degrees.
Figure 7.22: Incomplete RBBB; axis 25 degrees.

Chapter 8

Figure 8.6: LVH by voltage criteria and a typical strain pattern; axis 57 degrees.

Figure 8.7: RVH with an R-to-S ratio in lead V_1 of >1.0, RAD, normal QRS duration, and a strain pattern in the limb leads with the tallest QRS; axis 100 degrees.

Chapter 9

Figure 9.21: Acute anterior wall STEMI showing ST elevation in V_1–V_5 and in aVL with reciprocal depression in leads II, III, and aVF; axis is approximately 60 degrees.

Figure 9.22: Acute inferolateral wall STEMI showing ST elevation in leads II, III, and aVF, and in V_5 and V_6. Reciprocal depression is present in leads V_1–V_3 and in aVL. Early Q waves are present in leads III and aVF; axis is approximately 15 degrees.

Figure 9.23: Acute inferior wall STEMI showing ST elevation in II, III, and aVF, with reciprocal depression in leads I and aVL. Pathologic Q wave formation is incomplete. Axis is approximately 90 degrees.

Figure 9.24: Extensive acute anterior wall STEMI showing ST elevation in V_1–V_6 and in aVL. Pathologic Q waves are present in leads V_1–V_3. Reciprocal depression is present in all three inferior leads. Artifact has run lead I off the tracing. Axis is approximately 55 degrees.

Figure 9.25: Residual ST elevation with upward convexity and T wave inversion in the anterior wall compatible with an evolving non–Q wave anterior wall infarction. Note, however, that there is diminished R wave progression across the precordium. Axis is approximately 30 degrees.

Chapter 10

Figure 10.9: Nonspecific ST and T wave changes with sagging ST segments <1 mm deep and not clearly diagnostic of ischemia. Axis is approximately 42 degrees.

Figure 10.10: Horizontal or slightly downsloping ST depression of up to 2 mm, and an abrupt angle with the T wave, which are all characteristic of myocardial ischemia. There is poor R wave progression in leads V_1–V_3, raising the question of, but not proving, an old anterior infarction. Axis is approximately 36 degrees.

Figure 10.11: Sagging ST segments in many limb leads but fairly clear straight and horizontal or downsloping depression in leads V_4–V_6 of >1 mm, compatible with myocardial ischemia. Axis is approximately 40 degrees.

Figure 10.12: Full 12-lead tracing, again, with widespread ST depression reaching characteristic criteria for myocardial ischemia, most clearly in leads II and V_6. There is J point elevation in V_2 and V_3, but it is not characteristic of acute anterior wall infarction. Axis is approximately 0 degrees.

Index

Printed in the United States of America